THE ACTIVE POINTS TEST

of related interest

Pocket Handbook of Particularly Effective Acupoints for Common Conditions Illustrated in Color
Guo Changqing Guoyan and Zhaiwei Liu Naigang
ISBN 978 1 84819 120 4
eISBN 978 0 85701 094 0

Pocket Handbook of Body Reflex Zones Illustrated in Color
Guo Changqing Guoyan and Zhaiwei Liu Naigang
ISBN 978 1 84819 119 8
eISBN 978 0 85701 095 7

Meridians and Acupoints
Edited by Zhu Bing and Wang Hongcai
Advisor: Cheng Xinnong
ISBN 978 1 84819 037 5
eISBN 978 0 85701 021 6

Acupuncture Therapeutics
Edited by Zhu Bing and Wang Hongcai
Advisor: Cheng Xinnong
ISBN 978 1 84819 039 9
eISBN 978 0 85701 018 6

Eight Extraordinary Channels – Qi Jing Ba Mai
A Handbook for Clinical Practice and Nei Dan Inner Meditation
Dr David Twicken DOM, LAC
ISBN 978 1 84819 148 8
eISBN 978 0 85701 137 4

Developing Internal Energy for Effective Acupuncture Practice
Zhan Zhuang, Yi Qi Gong and the Art of Painless Needle Insertion
Ioannis Solos
ISBN 978 1 84819 183 9
eISBN 978 0 85701 144 2

The Compleat Acupuncturist
A Guide to Constitutional and Conditional Pulse Diagnosis
Peter Eckman
ISBN 978 1 84819 198 3
eISBN 978 0 85701 152 7

THE ACTIVE POINTS TEST

A Clinical Test for Identifying and Selecting Effective
Points for Acupuncture and Related Therapies

STEFANO MARCELLI

FOREWORDS BY DR DAVID ALIMI
AND DR IOAN DUMITRESCU

With *The Active Points Test in Auricular Puncture* by Marco Romoli
Translated from the Italian by Kim Pellitteri

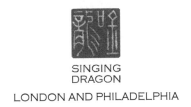

SINGING
DRAGON
LONDON AND PHILADELPHIA

The excerpt on pages 104–5 by Marco Romoli has been reproduced with the author's kind permission. The excerpt from Introduzione Pratica all'Auricolopuntura on pages 139–40 by Paul Nogier has been reproduced with kind permission of Éditions SATAS, Belgium and Libreria Cortina Torino srl. Figures 1.1–1.3, 2.1, 2.6–2.8, 2.11–2.18, 2.22, 3.1–3.4, 3.8–3.13, 3.16, 3.19–3.21, 5.2, 5.3, 5.7, 5.8 and 6.1 illustrated by Emanuel Montini; Figures 2.2–2.5, 2.21, 3.15, 3.17, 5.1 and 5.4–5.6 illustrated by Massimo Facchini; Figures 2.19 and 2.20 illustrated by Ioan F. Dumitrescu; Figures 4.1–4.3 illustrated by Salvatore Marcelli; Figures A.1–A.6 illustrated by Marco Romoli and Figures 3.7 and 3.15 illustrated by Massimo Facchini and Stefano Marcelli; all reproduced with permission. All other figures are the author's own or in the public domain.

This edition published in 2015
by Singing Dragon
an imprint of Jessica Kingsley Publishers
73 Collier Street
London N1 9BE, UK
and
400 Market Street, Suite 400
Philadelphia, PA 19106, USA

www.singingdragon.com

First published as *Il Test dei Punti Attivi* by Hoepli in 2010.

Copyright © Stefano Marcelli 2015
Forewords copyright © David Alimi and Ioan Florin Dumitrescu 2015

Library of Congress Cataloging in Publication Data
A CIP catalog record for this book is available from the Library of Congress

British Library Cataloguing in Publication Data
A CIP catalogue record for this book is available from the British Library

ISBN 978 1 84819 233 1
eISBN 978 0 85701 207 4

Printed and bound in Great Britain

For Anna, Francesca and Gabriel

To my patients and students

CONTENTS

LIST OF FIGURES AND TABLES

FIGURES

TABLES

FOREWORD

Writing the foreword to a work of such importance is a rare privilege and I thank Dr Marcelli for conceding me this honour. Acupuncture is an ancestral technique, transmitted according to the canons of Chinese medical tradition, which has been inherited through a powerful capacity of observation, associated with a cosmogonic conception.

Integrating, practising, experimenting and observing with a critical eye the patients' reactions to acupuncture manoeuvres is worthy of a great clinician such as Dr Stefano Marcelli is.

The 'Active Points Test' is the result of long experience. It is an original work in which the author shares with us his analytical deductions on the semiological values of clinical functional concordance in acupuncture. We discover that 'active points', both in traditional or auricular acupuncture and in reflex therapies generally, are precisely correlated to the intensity modulation of the symptoms of the pathology to be treated, especially in pain, while the point is being explored.

I want to say that on the neurophysiological plane this is perfectly explainable and it is also one of the fundamental notions we have been teaching our students for a long time. Neurological connections of capture, transport and management of the information obey certain laws, all formulated to converge toward maintaining the best possible homeostasis. This need depends strictly on the specificity of action potentials at the origin of the signals whose destination is the encephalon.

One of these great laws is Otto Kahler's and Arnold Pick's: at the level of every dermatome and respective vertical (3 above and 7 below) and horizontal connections, all informational fluxes converge toward the same neural unit (sensitive, motorial and autonomic), in order to synchronise all physiologies.

These physiologies obtain their passport in relation to the nature and intensity of the transported pathologies, of which the amplitude and frequency of action potentials are the reflex.

The described cybernetic mechanisms are subjected to precise priorities (sensitive, sensorial, motor and autonomic), with the aim of preserving the great homeostatic balance of our organism (the law of specific nervous energies, Hilton's law, Hebb's law, etc.).

During his important verification, Dr Stefano Marcelli has succeeded in objectifying the body of these intimate mechanisms by means of an attentive and methodical clinical observation of the practice of acupuncture and reflex therapies. This will contribute to the enrichment of their scientific basis.

Using a clear, didactic style, appropriate quotes and very effective iconography, he has given us a treasure in terms of clinical data which will be invaluable for the experienced practitioner and the student at his or her first practice. I hope this work will bring him gratitude and happiness.

Dr David Alimi[a]
Paris, France, 19 August 2009

a   Medical doctor, neurophysiologist. Adjunct Professor at the Faculty of Medicine at Bobigny, Paris 13; Chief of University Auricular Therapy Diplomas. As a researcher at the Gustave Roussy Institute of Cancer in Villejuif, he was the first to apply functional magnetic resonance to the study of auricular therapy.

FOREWORD TO THE
FIRST EDITION

I was surprised but happy to be invited by Dr Stefano Marcelli to say a few words to introduce his book, *The Active Points Test*. I will try to explain the reason for my mixed reaction.

First of all, I am happy to see that modern acupuncture is making clear progress. Italy, a country where a few decades ago I found numerous sources of inspiration when I made my debut in the field of cutaneous electrophysiology research (and if I had to limit myself to mentioning just one text, I would cite Fernando Ormea's monumental book *La cute organo di senso*), remains at the forefront in the research and application of modern reflex therapy. I was also happy to be recognised as a forerunner in cutaneous electrophysiology research and its application, which has resulted in my being given the honour of writing the preface to this book. But I am also happy to discover that not all the new conceptions about parallel medicine are the same, which in essence translates as a coming together towards the 'one great medicine' that unites us across the centuries. We could formulate an axiom, which would be paradoxical for geometry but real for medicine, to the effect that 'parallel lines can touch each other'.

I felt surprised because, as a supporter of technological testing who has always been faced with elaborate demonstrations, I found myself face to face with an original method, brilliant in its simplicity and effectiveness, which I hope will stand the test of time.

It is not up to me to judge or to give a verdict, but I can, however, encourage any creative initiative that leads to scientific progress in this very exciting field. I am faced with the dilemma of knowing that as a human being my powers are limited by the fact that I have not had sufficient time to observe Dr Marcelli closely, but I feel obliged to encourage him on this path. Dear Reader, you should commit to following him as well.

The work speaks for itself. It is aimed at all of our colleagues that are able to perform reflex therapy so that they may choose and test the effectiveness of the active points used in a wide range of therapeutic techniques.

So that I might better understand Dr Marcelli's personality, I asked if I could appraise some of his books from the bibliography indicated by him. Once received, I read them with care and pleasure. I felt profound admiration for his concise and clear style, for the coherence and continuity of his thought processes, in which a physiological and physiopathological interpretation is always present, and for the modern way in which his writing is organised.

So, in writing the preface to his book *The Active Points Test*, I cannot help but warmly recommend to the reader that he or she make the acquaintance of not just one of Dr Marcelli's works, but of a body of work that can already be described as a collection.

Dr Ioan Florin Dumitrescu (1937–1999)
Ronchin, France, 5 September 1994

PREFACE

The hope expressed by Dr Ioan Florin Dumitrescu in the preface to the first edition in 1994 that the Active Points Test might stand the test of time has been partially fulfilled. Twenty years after it was first published and 23 years since its creation, the time has come again for the Test to be presented to the reading public.

Validated in hundreds of cases since its first issue, the Active Points Test has not changed fundamentally. A few small changes, which were already creeping in at the time of the first edition, have been made to simplify the procedure and make it accessible to anyone dealing with illness and with pain and functional impotence in particular.

It is not, therefore, necessary to be an acupuncturist or to have a degree in medicine or surgery to understand and perform the Test. Physiotherapists, kinesiologists, chiropractors, osteopaths, practitioners of shiatsu and tuina, fascia manipulators and experts in every kind of massage, including followers of Rolf and Dicke, provided they have the enthusiasm required to learn and to treat patients, can all use the Active Points Test to enrich their own disciplines.

In the first edition I paid particular attention to gathering data so that my work might be called scientific, within the poor limitations of this word, and produced a clinical-statistical study through evidence-based medicine. In this second edition, I have focused on describing the Active Points Test in the clearest way possible through experience-based medicine.

Enjoy your work,

Stefano Marcelli
Darfo Boario Terme

Chapter 1

THE TEST

1.1 DEFINITION AND PARTICULARS

The *Active Points Test* is a clinical, manual and instrumental test for evaluating the therapeutic potential of cutaneous stimulation.

It is based on the discovery of *the latent awareness of the active point*: the realisation that a patient with an ongoing symptom can be made aware of the capacity of a few points and areas of skin to treat his or her discomfort, so that the patient takes part in the diagnosis and in the neuroreflex therapy.

Manual pinching or *contact with an acupuncture needle* (Figure 1.1, page 22) or with the nib of a ballpoint pen (see Figure 2.9, page 45) on certain points of the skin *immediately* reduces or neutralises most ongoing symptoms, showing itself to be an extremely reliable test (96.15%) for evaluating *a priori* the effectiveness of manual or needle therapy, whether it is western in origin, such as mesotherapy, auricular puncture, neural therapy and physiotherapy, or of oriental origin, like acupuncture, shiatsu and tuina.

The Active Points Test consists in stimulating the skin to the appropriate degree, after asking the patient to notify any change in perception of the symptom from which he or she is suffering. Therefore, for the execution of the Test it is necessary and indispensable *for the symptom to be clearly perceptible*. The range of symptoms for which the Test can be used is vast, from articular pain (Traditional Chinese Medicine's *Bi* syndrome) to migraine, from nasal obstruction to tachycardia, and even for borderline cases of asthenia and depression (see Table 1.1, page 26). During this exposition, particularly in the practical section, I will often make reference to pain and functional impotence, since these are the most frequently observed symptoms.

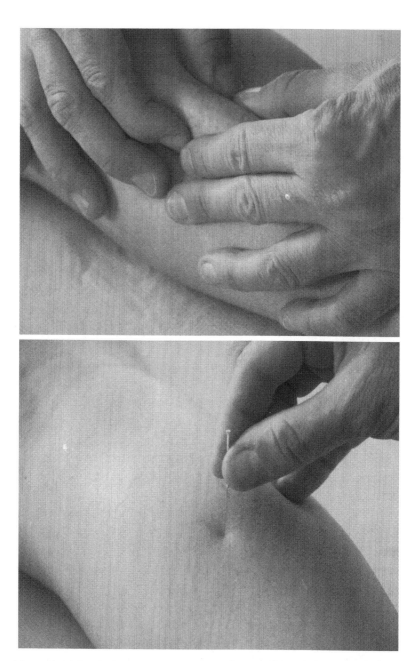

Figure 1.1 The Active Points Test executed manually and then with the point of an acupuncture needle on point BL-57 Chengshan of the Bladder Channel

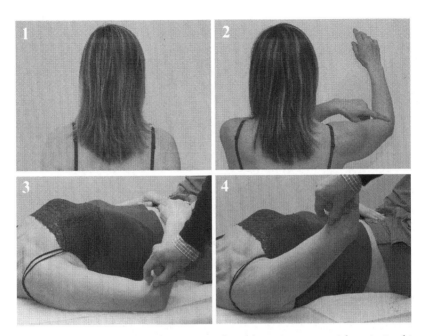

Figure 1.2 The Active Points Test performed on a patient with pain in the elbow which appears when the arm is raised, irrespective of posture
(1) At rest. (2) Arm raised and subsequent appearance of symptom. (3) Identification of most painful local point, corresponding to acupuncture point LI-11 Quchi. (4) Test during the movement.

The Active Points Test costs nothing and requires little time and the minimum amount of equipment. Since an ounce of experience is worth more than a hundred years of theory, here are a few everyday examples:

- An office worker has a pain in his shoulder which torments him day and night, in all positions.

- A woman gets a twinge in her wrist every time she turns the key in the lock, wrings out the washing or grips a bottle to pour a drink.

- A business manager experiences a stinging sensation in the buttock after sitting in a car for ten minutes.

- A climbing enthusiast notices a pain in his elbow when he grabs hold of a rock spur to continue his climb.

- A marathon runner complains that her heel, which she cannot set down without feeling pain, is threatening to interrupt her sporting career.

- A labourer would like to be free of the continuous stomach ache which no ordinary treatment has managed to overcome.

- A shop assistant cannot find a remedy for a chronic cough which sets in when she takes deep breaths.

Irrespective of the core diagnosis: muscular contraction, articular inflammation, tendonitis, neuralgia or any other, a few points of the skin will be subjected to the Active Points Test, either alleviating or neutralising the symptom (Figure 1.2, page 23). Near to or away from the seat of the symptom, the skin will be pinched between the thumb and forefinger of one or both hands, or contact will be made with the point of a needle or the nib of an empty ballpoint pen, or with the aid of a glass stick or massager for the points of the ears, searching for a particularly painful point. The patient will then be asked if the pain provoked by these actions alleviates or neutralises the original pain: the one that motivated him or her to seek a consultation.

1.2 INDICATIONS FOR AND LIMITATIONS OF THE TEST

Indications for the Active Points Test are symptoms, both continuing and ongoing, *which are clearly perceptible* to the patient. First of all, these are predominantly *locoregional* affections: muscular, articular and nerve pain, extra-articular, somatic or visceral pain which is easily pinpointed (by sinusitis, phlebitis, or gastritis), irritations of the motor or sensory functions such as regional pruritus (e.g. vaginal, anal) or tinnitus. The Test may also be indicated for symptoms which present periodically, but only if they are regular and close together.

I have also subjected to the Test a few cases of asthenia and psychosomatic tension, some cases of dermatological pathology accompanied by pruritus and pain, and a few cases involving an irritating creaking in the joints (see Figure 3.20, page 113), all with good results. There is, however, no reason why the Test should not also be indicated for other affections of a general nature, as long as the symptoms are clearly perceptible to the patient. The only limitations of the Test are found in cases where it is impossible to obtain information from the patient as to the effectiveness of manual or needle stimulation.

We cannot rule out the idea that an extremely sensitive patient might derive an immediate benefit from the stimulation of a few points, even when suffering from sideropenic anaemia, 'endogenous' depression or other systemic affections.

Table 1.1 (page 26) gives a reasoned list of the indications for performing the Active Points Test which, as well as being a test for the evaluation *a priori* of the therapeutic potential of some points on the skin, may also provide indications for the exclusion of some therapies which are based on the stimulation of those points. In the few cases where I ascertained such a condition – *absolute non-responders* – acupuncture brought no benefit, and in some cases even caused a temporary deterioration of the symptomatology. A systematic analysis of other reflex therapy maps might, however, reduce the number of cases which do not respond to the Test.

1.3 THERAPIES FOR WHICH THE TEST IS USEFUL

The Active Points Test is a diagnostic test which does not pertain exclusively to one particular methodology, and may be used advantageously in all puncture therapies and in those manual therapies whose objective is the treatment of pain and functional impotence and other ongoing symptoms. Table 1.2 (see page 26) shows a list, albeit not exhaustive, of therapies which could make the Active Points Test part of their diagnostic armament.

TABLE 1.1 THE ACTIVE POINTS TEST INDICATIONS

All continuing and ongoing symptoms			
Pain	somatic visceral	spontaneous	
		induced	kinetic positional palpatory
Esthesic irritations other than pain	pruritus burning/stinging sensation swelling paresthesias noise (e.g. tinnitus, creaking of the joints)		
Functional limitation to various systems	respiratory	nasal obstruction, rhinorrhea, cough, dysphonia, aphonia, hiccups, dyspnoea	
	digestive	dysphagia, nausea, vomiting, spasms, feeling of heaviness or knotting	
	locomotive	muscle contracture, limitation and blockage of movement, articular noises, sense of unsteadiness	
	genito-urinary	dysuria, tension, heaviness	
	cardiovascular	alterations in rhythm, palpitation, symptoms of hypotension and hypertension	

TABLE 1.2 THERAPIES THAT BENEFIT FROM
THE ACTIVE POINTS TEST

Manual Techniques	Puncture Techniques
Shiatsu	Acupuncture
Tuina	Auricular puncture
Physiotherapy	Mesotherapy
Applied Kinesiology	Neural therapy
Chiropractice	Cranial puncture
Osteopathy	Hand and foot puncture
Rolfing	Nasal puncture
Deep-tissue massage	Facial injection therapy
Fascia therapy	Puncture of the oral mucosa

I.4 AN *EX ADIUVANTIBUS* CRITERION

In clinical practice, when there are insufficient diagnostic elements to allow for the use of logical deductive reasoning to orient therapy, recourse is made to the *ex adiuvantibus* criterion. This is a kind of preliminary to the treatment which gives a clear indication as to whether a drug or any other therapeutic defence is effective against the ongoing pathology. What doctor, physiotherapist, shiatsu or tuina practitioner, or western masseur, during the course of his/her practice, has never said these words: 'Let's try this – a drug, a muscular exercise, a nutritional supplement – and see what happens'?

The Active Points Test is, therefore, a proper *ex adiuvantibus* criterion for choosing an effective remedy. It gives us the opportunity to find out in advance if the points we intend to use, chosen in accordance with one of the many existing methods of stimulation of the cutis, will have a therapeutic effect or not. Its theoretical assumptions are no different from those of the usual laboratory tests, whose purpose is to orient the diagnosis and specify the therapy to be used. It is similar to allergy tests carried out to check the way the body reacts to certain substances, and on the basis of which a specific therapy is determined. A stronger analogy can be made between the Active Points Test and the antibiogram, performed on a biological sample infected by a bacterial strain, in order to determine, from a fairly wide-ranging list, the most effective antibiotic molecules for combating its development in the body.

I.5 KINESIOLOGY AND APPLIED KINESIOLOGY

The first name given to the Active Points Test was the *Acupuncture Kinesiologic Test*,[1] because of its formal similarity with the muscle tests used in Applied Kinesiology. Saudelli included it under this name among the techniques of *Touch Localization* from the same discipline.[2]

Briefly, kinesiology (from the Greek *kínesis* = movement) is the branch of physiology which studies the movement of muscles. The areas to which it can be applied are the pathology of the musculoskeletal system and the relationship between the latter's organs and the nervous system. The most modern version, called *Applied Kinesiology*, envisages special diagnostic manoeuvres based on a test for evaluating muscle strength.

The kinesiologist manually weighs up the strength of a given muscle, defining it as *strong* or *weak*, after which one of the special movements is performed. Then the strength of that muscle is tested again to see if the movement has caused any changes, either by weakening a strong muscle or strengthening a weak one (Figure 1.3). If the strength of a weak muscle increases, the movement will be considered useful for therapy; vice versa if it weakens a strong muscle, it will provide a clue to the cause of the disease. The movements are various and can relate to factors which are either internal or external to the patient. The muscle test can be performed in order to discover if a substance (homeopathic remedy, food, synthetic drug, etc.) will lead to an increase in the strength of the muscle tested and whether it may be used advantageously in therapy. If, on the other hand, it leads to a weakening in muscle strength, it will be considered indirect proof of an allergy or intolerance. Moreover, the muscle test is used to discover whether a point or area of the body, or the nerve segments or energy channels of acupuncture, has any influence on muscle strength and consequently, if they should be stimulated during therapy (touch localization).

For example, after testing the strength of the humeral biceps and defining it as strong, the patient may be invited to touch the appendicular point with the index finger of his or her other hand. During the movement, the muscle is tested again and if it proves to be weaker, the limb will be presumed to be suffering from a chronic problem which is not evident, but which is capable of having a negative effect on the patient's health. The allergic *potential* of some foods or the therapeutic capacity of food supplements can be evaluated in a similar manner. Speciani, during research into food allergies, computerised and tried to objectify the muscle test by connecting the patient's femoral quadriceps to a dynamometer, so as to evaluate the change in muscle strength after administering certain foods and other diluted substances under the tongue. For further information, see basic texts on classical and Applied Kinesiology.[3,4] The views of Stephen Barrett (retired psychiatrist), who accuses kinesiology of charlatanry, and of Tim Bolen (lawyer) who counter-accuses him of falsehood and conspiracy, are curious.[5]

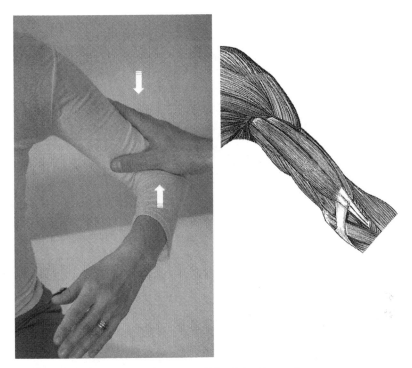

Figure 1.3 Applied Kinesiology test of the deltoid muscle
The patient tries to raise her arm while the therapist blocks it. The function of the
muscle test is to define a particular muscle as *strong* or *weak* in order to evaluate
the variations in its strength after special movements.

As in Applied Kinesiology muscle tests, the Active Points Test also
directly correlates the patient's symptom and his/her immediate
response to the therapeutic activity on the point being tested. The
fundamental difference resides in the fact that in the Active Points Test
the patient is included in the Test. In actual fact, as a 'living sensitive
cybernetic machine', the patient's immediate responses through
stimulated nerve signals let us know whether the point being explored
is 'active' in terms of regulating the *symptom – therapy – reduction of
symptom* circle, and is to be treated.

1.6 OTHER TESTS IN ACUPUNCTURE

As well as traditional analysis of the radial pulses and Kenyon's
experimental attempt to objectify it through an oscillographic

recording,[6] two other tests exist which evaluate the energy state of certain points and the energy channels to which they belong. Their execution presents, however, certain practical difficulties.

Electroacupuncture according to Voll (EAV) is a method of measuring the electrical resistance of acupuncture points.[7,8] Variations between too much and too little resistance, and a phenomenon known as *a fall in the index*, reveal the pathological states of organs which the acupoints are thought to guard. Due to the high number of points in existence, electropuncture analysis is only carried out on those situated in the corners of the nails on the hands and feet, for a total of 40 readings. The other test, also performed on the *jing* points, the corners of the nails, goes by the name of its inventor: *Akabane's Test*. In practice, the patient's resistance to heat is measured with a stick of moxa. The lighted tip of the stick is moved repeatedly, sometimes using a small supporting device, between the *jing* point of the channel to be tested and the centre of the nail. This is called the *Meridian Imbalance Dolorimeter.* A reduction in resistance, measured by the number of times the stick has to be moved before the patient feels pain instead of heat, indicates an excess of energy in the corresponding channel, while the opposite, that is to say an increase in resistance, indicates a state of emptiness. Kazuko Itaya and Yoshio Manata perfected an electronic radiating device for the optimal execution of Akabane's test.[9,10] Although potentially useful, these tests do not offer the chance to find out 'immediately' the extent to which the point examined is related to the patient's current disorder and therefore valid for therapeutic purposes.

1.7 THE ACUPUNCTURE ENERGY SYSTEM

As the Active Points Test originated in the field of acupuncture, it is opportune to set out the general considerations that contributed to its creation.

The acupuncture energy system, with its points and channels, can be compared to a complex communications network with lines underground, above ground and in the air, and equipped with railway stations, airports, junctions and crossroads of varying importance. Working on acupoints is like managing traffic on the network, increasing and decreasing its intensity and frequency. Some points are as central and strategically important to the system as the railway stations in Paris and the airports in London are to Europe. Others are less important and are capable only of influencing small parts of a single route. According to the doctrine of the Qi in Traditional Chinese Medicine (TCM), there are some energy lines whose flow is more or less constant through time and relatively independent of the seasons (the Extraordinary Channels), and some lines which are under the dominion of seasonal, meteorological and cosmic energies (the Principal Channels). This is comparable to the frequency of buses for commuting students being increased in autumn or special trains for the most popular holiday destinations being inserted into timetables in summer. Then there are airports from where aircraft depart to distant regions, creating fast and direct connections that do not affect the overland and underground lines. This is the case with the *opening points* which activate the Extraordinary Channels. From this comparison it is easy to understand how slight alterations to the energy state of some important points can influence traffic on the whole network, while the effect of even serious disturbances at other peripheral or secondary points is indifferent in terms of the general economy of the system. Therefore, if we consider disease as an acute or chronic alteration of the energy system, it is ever more necessary to identify the stations, that is to say the best points, where to intervene to restore the original balance to the system. Chinese energy doctrine, with its numerous philosophical categories and the immense cosmological culture to which it refers, hardly lends itself to a *simple solution* to the problems that are presented daily to those who practise acupuncture. Even an expert can end up applying pre-packaged suggestions and points prescriptions which, while on the one hand are extremely useful and effective with regard to symptoms and diseases that would clear up spontaneously over time, may be completely unsuitable or inadequate for diseases with a complex and original symptomology which tend to be chronic. The knowledge and choice of local points in certain affections, such as those of a locoregional nature, require only an accurate study of the points on the channels that cross the affected region. The choice of points which are far from the seat of the disease is more complicated and unfruitful, yet these are the points which Traditional Chinese Medicine defines as 'causal' and more important for the purposes of a radical therapy.

Being aware of my limits in the difficult application of the diagnostic methods of Traditional Chinese Medicine was one of the driving forces behind the creation of a quick and effective method for determining the most suitable local and distant points for treating the majority of affections encountered in daily practice. For further information, see classical and modern texts about acupuncture and related techniques.[11,12,13,14,15,16,17,18]

1.8 THE DIFFICULTIES OF ACUPUNCTURE

No acupuncturist or reflex therapist, however prepared or conscientious he or she may be, can deny that the study of Traditional Chinese Medicine's energy system presents considerable difficulties, whether on a theoretical plane or a practical one. The theoretical difficulties pertain to the concept of the Qi, an energetic entity which, although in part explained through its electrical manifestations (electrodermal points, electrical channels),[19] can still not be proved absolutely nor reproduced, due to its subdivision between the *Yin* and *Yang* poles, its energy currents and the intricate links between internal organs and superficial paths which it has at its disposal. The education of a graduate in western medicine is largely concentrated on the physio-chemical aspects of the body's functions, and the image the graduate is left with at the end of his or her studies is that of a 'machine' which, if compared to modern achievements in robotic engineering, is rather 'imperfect'. If we then discuss diagnosis through examination of the patient's physiognomy, looking at the tongue and taking the radial pulses, the difficulties appear insurmountable. This is why the doctrinal system on which acupuncture is based cannot be rejected *a priori* by those whose observations are based principally on facts from the physical and chemical world.

Doctors involved in acupuncture belong to two distinct categories. In the first are the followers of neurology, who understand and accept the neurophysiology argument about stimulation induced by puncture; in the second category are the ranks of mystics and those disillusioned by the ineffectiveness of academic medicine on the quality of life. To these can be added the doctors who try to reflect more objectively on the constitution of living beings and of man in particular, and who have supplemented their university studies with philosophical, religious and esoteric texts. These people, especially if they are practitioners of traditional acupuncture, are in the same mental state as those who believe in the existence of life after death and adapt their behaviour to a morality that corresponds to their beliefs, convinced that sooner or later they will succeed in unveiling the mystery.

The practical difficulties (Table 1.3) are a direct consequence of those theories, as the therapeutic movements in acupuncture are completely blind to the points and to the energy paths over which the former are supposed to be situated.

TABLE 1.3 COMPOSITION OF
ACUPUNCTURE MERIDIAN SYSTEM

Over 1000 classified points	between ordinary (670) and extra (387), of which at least 50 are in current use.
Approximately 50 energy routes	(Principal Channels, Extraordinary Channels, Luo, Secondary and minor Luo).
At least 10 points	endowed with therapeutic activity traditionally or 'scientifically' accepted for any affliction or symptom.

Chapter 2

PRACTICE

2.1 INITIAL QUESTION

The Active Points Test is the fruit of a few observations made in fortuitous circumstances, following a process of intellectual speculation which lasted at least three years.

Around 1990 I began to wonder why quite different therapies for pain and functional impotence had the same satisfactory results. For eight years I had been a practitioner of mesotherapy, acupuncture, auricular puncture and neural therapy, often in combination. Occasionally I had turned to Tens and IR laser therapy and had been racking my brains to find a valid criterion for deciding when to use one or the other, whether to choose a simple needle or microinjection with anaesthetic, with or without adding an anti-inflammatory. After much reflection, I believed I had identified the common link between my therapies, or at least those related to puncture, as the homeopathic principle.[20] After all, I thought, when a painful area is punctured, an artificial pain is being applied cutaneously to a spot which is already suffering from one that is a pathological and subcutaneous. For this reason, therapy based on puncture, even without drugs, respects the axiom of homeopathy – 'cure like with like'. Doubt remained (and still does) as to whether a gesture, rather than infinitessimal doses of a substance, could be considered homeopathy. To this end, the work carried out by Weihe and his students on the correlation between homeopathic remedies and painful points on the body is of interest.[21] With regard to mesotherapy (punctures + anaesthetic + other drugs), which I was lucky enough to have been introduced to some time before by excellent teachers,[22,23,24] I had noticed that cocktails containing the most painful drugs (vitamin B12 and chlorproethazine) were far and away the most effective.

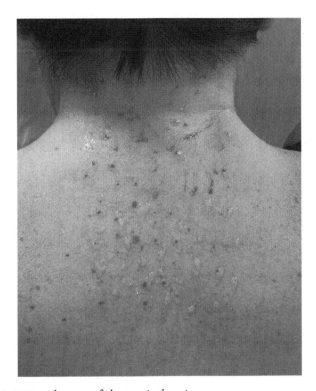

Figure 2.1 Mesotherapy of the cervical region
Therapeutic bleeding incidental to the execution of the *nappage* technique.

It was my opinion that simultaneous punctures with multi-injectors and repeated punctures from *nappage*,[25,26] sometimes with profuse bleeding (Figure 2.1), had an effect which went beyond that of the drugs.[27] During my acupuncture training, I had come across teachers who were 'heavy-handed' but acknowledged as very good. I remembered Roccia boasting that the cutaneous infiltration of a few drops of distilled water on the abdominal projection points of the ureter was decisive.[28] Roccia also referred to the astonishing recoveries achieved by Head and MacKenzie through the application of mustard plaster to the reflex skin pain (dermatalgia) of stomach pathologies.[b] In early mesotherapy, Pistor predicted the use of 'induced pain' in rebellious

---

b   Revulsive poultices prepared from mustard seed flour, cooked and wrapped in gauze. The term 'revulsion' indicated a dilation of the cutaneous blood vessels for the purpose of decongesting the internal organs.

cases.[c] The effects of neural therapy, based solely on injections of the anaesthetic procaine,[29,30] also seemed logical to me. What confused me, though, was how both pain induced by mesotherapy or acupuncture, and neural therapy anaesthesia, which are complete opposites, could have a beneficial effect. Furthermore, leaving aside personal issues, I noticed that every day masseurs, massotherapists, physiotherapists and shiatsu practitioners (tuina was still unknown in Italy) were just as successful at treating pain using methods which were different from my own. At the same time, persistently and with varying results, orthopaedists, physiatrists, rheumatologists and anaesthetists were injecting cortisone into shoulders, elbows, wrists, knees and ankles. During that period, oxygen-ozone injections were also beginning to be mentioned in the field of antalgy. The question remained: was the recovery or improvement brought about by all of these therapies due to injections of anti-inflammatories, to anaesthetic, to simple, multiple or simultaneous punctures, to stimulation from massage, to bleeding or to something else?

2.2 FINAL OBSERVATIONS

In 1993 I arrived at my final observations, thanks to which I realised that the only factor common to these therapies was that they all involved the cutis. Massages and the *palper rouler* technique in particular, simple, multiple or repeated punctures, injections of drugs and anaesthetic (including cortisone injections), 'pass through' areas of skin that are, anatomically, closely connected to the pain experienced by the patient.

The crucial observation was made when I started practising acupuncture. When I was studying the functions of points, in the concluding section of the book *The Foundations of Acupuncture and Traditional Chinese Medicine* dedicated to the therapeutic properties of some of the major points,[31] I had found the following indication relating to point ST-38 Tiaokou (Figure 2.2) on the Stomach Channel:

---

c   'Currently in Mesotherapy, when we have to treat a disease in which pain has for a long time been the most important element in the clinical picture, if the cocktails which are usually effective have not been successful, we will turn to these short stimulations which, in many difficult cases, give unexpected positive results. To do this we use the multi-injector to distribute distilled water based cocktails, which are painful injections' (Pistor, note 22, p.55).

Special point for acute shoulder problems. The needle is inserted in the direction of Chengshan (BL-57), *strong manipulation is performed and the patient is requested to move the shoulder during treatment.*

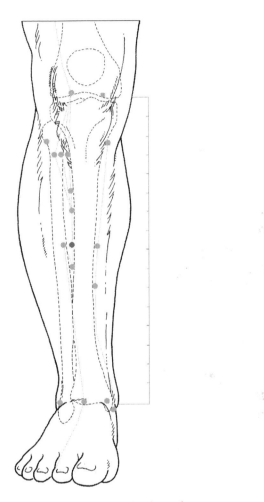

Figure 2.2 Point ST-38 Tiaokou on the Stomach Channel

The particular nature of the method had stuck in my mind, because the patient was invited to participate, to help the doctor, just as he/ she is asked to clench his fist repeatedly so as to distend a vein in order for a blood sample to be taken, or to swallow during a gastroscopy to facilitate the insertion of the endoscope. Yet I had never considered using it because I had never seen it performed. The opportunity presented itself when I had a patient who was suffering from an acute pain in the shoulder, on which I had tried every treatment I knew without it having the slightest effect. Once the needle was in but before starting the prescribed manipulation, when I asked the patient to move his shoulder as was indicated in the manual, he replied that the pain had disappeared as if by magic. But how could it have done, if the needle had barely penetrated the skin?

After therapy, the patient left the surgery free of his problem and satisfied. I was astonished, and overcome by the fanatical enthusiasm of one who believes he has found the philosopher's stone. However, the fire of that emotion was soon put out by attempts to use the puncturing of the same point in successive cases of acute shoulder pain, as it proved effective in few of them. A retrospective study of the medical case histories, which I always take down very thoroughly, of those patients who had benefited from the puncture of Tiaokou, revealed that they were all suffering or had suffered from disturbances to the digestive system and, specifically, from functional gastroduodenal disorders, which explained the effectiveness of using a point belonging to the Stomach Channel.

Not long afterwards, when I was treating myself for neuralgia caused by a wisdom tooth, during the manipulation of the needles on the points I had chosen, I noticed that only one acted immediately to soothe my pain, the others having no effect at all. The point was ST-6 Jiache (Figure 2.3), 'by chance' on the Stomach Channel again, but this time right next to the tooth responsible and not far from the injury, unlike Tiaokou in relation to the shoulder. So it was the pain caused by the manipulation that was interfering with my pain and neutralising it, and not who knows what obscure principle. The next morning, when the sharp pains returned, I tried pinching the skin on point ST-6 Jiache between two fingers. It worked even without the needle puncture. It was not as effective, but the difference was negligible. It clicked at that moment that I could test how points would work before starting the therapy.

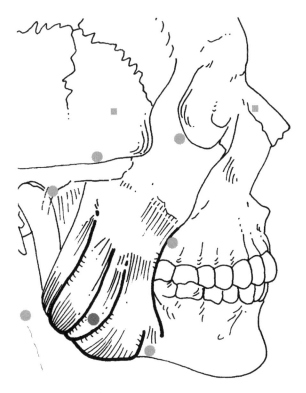

Figure 2.3 Point ST-6 Jiache

I began systematically to subject all my patients who I considered suitable for acupuncture, mesotherapy and neural therapy to the Test, which I initially called the *Acupuncture Kinesiologic Test*, because of its formal similarities with the *Touch Localization* of Applied Kinesiology. Shortly afterwards, I changed to the more ecumenical name of the Active Points Test.

In traditional acupuncture, SI-3 Houxi Small Intestine (Figure 2.4, page 40) and CV-24 Chengjiang Conception Vessel (Figure 2.5, page 40) are also used for an acute stiff neck, in the same way as Tiaokou is used for a painful shoulder. For acute lumbalgia beginning no earlier than 48 hours before treatment, GV-26 Renzhong is suggested and, even though I have never seen mention of it in books, in Nanjing in 1996 I was present at a needle manipulation in point ST-9 Renyin Stomach (Figure 2.5) to treat homolateral scialtalgia, while the patient flexed his calves with the aim of exacerbating the pain.

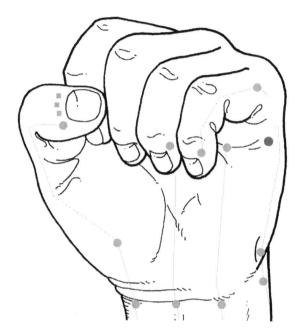

Figure 2.4 Point SI-3 Houxi

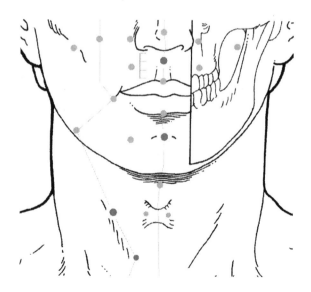

Figure 2.5 Points GV-26 Renzhong (labial sulcus), CV-24 Chengjiang (chin fold) and ST-9 Renyin (neck)

Instinctively, a doubt arose in my mind: was there an Active Points Test in acupuncture and traditional Chinese massage? If not, why hadn't it been invented? Was it perhaps because the ancient Chinese doctors did not understand the exact function of the nerves, or the cerebral substrate responsible for movement and consciousness? Was it perhaps because there was less interaction then between doctor and patient than exists now? Or was it perhaps because taking a case history was not considered a prerogative of TCM? Considering the surprising number of extraordinary points (see Figure 3.14 page 101),[14] it is possible that something similar to the Active Points Test was common practice, but that no one had thought to write it down for posterity's sake. Or else they had not needed to because some other form of information allowed them to 'see' the link between a painful shoulder and the Tiaokou point, between a stiff neck and the Houxi point, and so on.

2.3 ONE NAIL DRIVES OUT ANOTHER

Knowledge of Melzack and Wall's Gate control theory of pain was fundamental in the formulation of the Active Points Test.[32,33,34] The work of the two pioneers is well structured and stretches across several decades. It includes the neuroanatomy and neurophysiology of marrow and of the brain, pharmacology and psychology. The *Gate Control Theory of Pain* will be explored in depth in Chapter 4. In essence, it tells us that pain transmitted to the brain through fine, slow, unmyelinated A-delta (A∂), and C fibres (Table 2.1, page 42) is inhibited by the transmission of another stimulus, which could be a needle puncture or an intense heat, travelling along thicker, faster, myelinated A-beta (Aß) fibres. Metaphorically, it can be described as follows: two trains are travelling on different tracks towards the same destination. At some point along the way they find themselves on a single track. The stronger train (the therapy) will be the one to take over the track. The other train (the pain) will be made to queue or will be cancelled. Neurophysiology apart, the gate theory can be understood by everyone.

TABLE 2.1 SENSORY FIBRES AND CUTANEOUS RECEPTORS

Type	Diameter	Speed	Associated sensory receptors
Aß	6–12 μm	33–75 m/s	All cutaneous mechanoreceptors
A∂	1–5 μm	3–30 m/s	Free nerve endings for touch and pressure Thermoreceptors for cold Neospinothalamic tract nociceptors
C	0.2–1.5 μm	0.5–2.0 m/s	Paleospinothalamic tract nociceptors Thermoreceptors for warmth

If someone falls off their bicycle in the morning and sustains a *painful* bruise to the knee, and in the evening the same person also starts to suffer from a *very painful* pulpitis due to untreated tooth decay, the pain of the first injury will be cancelled out by the agony of the second. The famous Latin maxim *ubi maior minus cessat*, 'The weak capitulates before the strong', is also valid here. Bowing to popular wisdom, we can use the incisive proverb: 'One nail drives out another'. As for me, I do not believe that any pain exists that cannot be cancelled out, if only temporarily by the need to escape from a potentially fatal peril. One day many years ago, a very acute back pain had confined me to bed following a particularly exhausting tennis session. A sudden crash and an inhuman cry from my wife (it's all right, she is still alive!) brought me to my feet, curing me in an instant. A very brief but intense earth tremor had pulled a cupboard from its supports on the kitchen wall. Of course, my back pain was nothing serious and I was very determined to live. The history of medicine suggests that there was an excellent forerunner to Melzack and Wall, no less a person than Hippocrates (see Figure 2.6).

A careful observer of the sick and of illness, during the first century of our era he had written: 'When two pains appear contemporaneously but not in the same place, the most violent one will obscure the other.'[35]

Aphorifmus.   46.
Duorum dolorum qui fimul fiunt non fecundū
eundem locum,uehementior denigrat alterum.

The.   Si dolor geminus non eodem loco infeftat,qui uehe-
       mentior eft,alterum leuiorem obfcurat.

Leo.   Duobus doloribus fimul eundem locum infeftanti-
       bus,uehementior alterum obfcurat.

APHOR. 46.

Δύο πόνων ἅμα γινομένων μὴ κατὰ τὴν αὐ-
τὴν τόπιν, ὁ σφοδρότερ@· ἀμαυροῖ τὸν
ἕτερον.

Duobus doloribus non in eodem loco
obortis, vehementior alterum ob-
fcurabit.

Hic non folum dolores, fed quæcunque mor-
borum intelliguntur fymptomata. Doce-
mur ita, dolorem dolore, morbum morbo levari
interdum. An obnubilatur in mente perceptio
doloris levioris a vehementiore, quemadmo-
dum lumen minus obfcuratur a majore?

Figure 2.6 Images concerning Aphorism II / 46 of Hippocrates' Aphorisms,
taken from public domain books
Above: 'SUPER APHORISMOS IACOBI FORORIVENSIS ET GALENI
SUPER EISMOS COMMENTARIOS [...] VENETII APUD IUNTAS 1547'.
Below: 'HIPPOCRATIS COI APHORISMI NOTATIONIBUS VARIORUM
ILLUSTRATI. VOLUMEN I. JO. CHR. RIEGER. HAGAE COMITUM APUD
PETRUM VAN CLEEF 1607'.

2.4 MATERIALS

The Active Points Test requires above all the use of the hands, either
one or both, where tissue is 'pinchable' (Figure 2.7). However, where
it is not easy to lift a parcel of skin, such as on the skull, the fingers,
the palms, the soles of the feet, the ears and the nose, the glass stick
(Figure 2.8) or the nib of an empty biro will be used (Figure 2.9). The
latter will as a rule be used as an alternative to the specific massager
on the auricular points, since these are difficult to explore with larger
instruments. Those who are licensed to do so may use an acupuncture
needle (Figure 2.9).

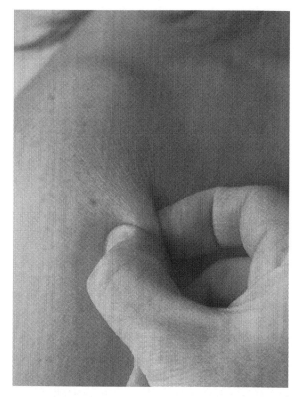

Figure 2.7 Pinching of loose skin
The Active Points Test carried out in relation to a spontaneous symptom (frozen shoulder).

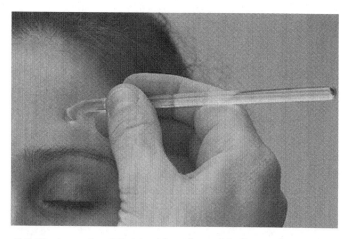

Figure 2.8 Testing point GB-14 with a glass stick (batôn de verre)

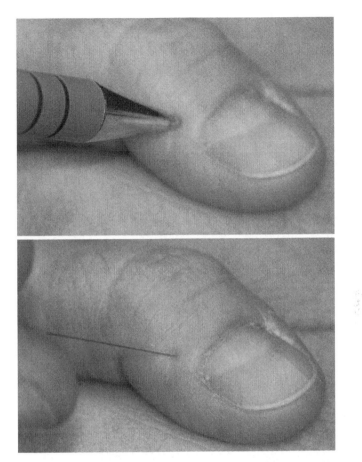

Figure 2.9 The Active Points Test using the nib of an empty biro and a needle on taut skin

A needle is definitely the most powerful instrument for testing how the active points are; however, many years' experience has taught me to look for and test points manually first and afterwards with a needle, for three reasons. The first follows in the footsteps of the old Chinese adage also mentioned by Cracolici (pp.174–175): 'In order to puncture a point well, you first need to knock and if this is done gently, the door will open.'

By pinching we prepare the patient for the pain of the puncture. The second reason is that pinching makes the area of the point larger and calls the Qi to the surface, a phenomenon also well known to acupuncture electrophysiology by the name fenestration – occlusion.[19]

Without exception, pinching the skin is more easily tolerated by the patient than puncture, and it also induces a more 'measurable' pain. Last, the hands, the stick, the massager and the biro nib never cause bleeding, which sometimes happens when points are tested with needles, and it is always a good idea to take precautions in order to avoid the risk of possible infection. When using needles, they should always be flexible and neither too long nor too short. Those measuring from 0.25 or 0.3 mm × 25 mm are the most indicated.

If the patient's skin is greasy or too dry and the fingers slip over it, especially during the execution of the Test in the presence of kinetic symptoms, it may be cleaned with an alcohol solution, or a slip of paper of around ten cm² cut from the couch linen may be held between the fingers (Figure 2.10).

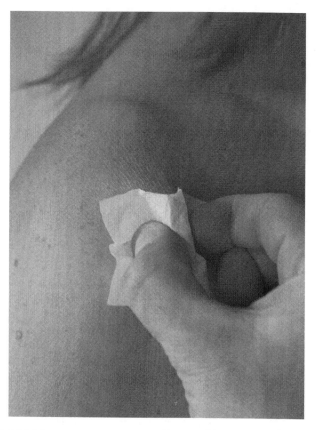

Figure 2.10 Using paper on greasy or slippery skin

2.5 CLEANING AND DISINFECTING THE SKIN

Washing your hands and cleaning the part of the skin to be searched for painful points is excellent practice. I do not need to write a treatise on it. I must stress one recommendation: if you are considering needle therapy after performing the Test (acupuncture, mesotherapy, neural therapy, etc), it is better to avoid using detergents or disinfectants which contain irritants or worse, essential oils, insofar as the needle, even during the Test, could carry potentially allergenic molecules into the derma and subcutaneous tissue. The molecules and disinfectant combinations are numerous. I personally use a solution of *clorexidine* and *benzalkonium chloride* as suggested by the French Mesotherapy Society, which is available today in many supermarkets. Let us not forget, too, that the tips of the glass stick and the auricular massager, and the nib of the biro, must always be disinfected after contact with the patient. Any needles used must be disposed of.

2.6 TEST PROCEDURE

The Active Points Test is to be carried out in accordance with a precise sequence of steps:

1. classification of the symptom
2. explanations and instructions to patient
3. search for painful points
4. execution of the Test.

1. Classification of the symptom

Once the pain, functional impotence or other symptom has been verified as *ongoing* and *continuous* (clearly perceptible),[d] it will be classified as follows:

- *spontaneous*, if it occurs and remains of its own accord, or
- *induced*, if it occurs in determined circumstances. It is characterised as:

---

d   The Test cannot be used for non-continuous symptoms, except for those occurring regularly and close together.

- *kinetic*, occurring during the execution of a movement

- *positional*, occurring when part or the whole of the body assumes a position[e] (laterally flexed neck, supination of hand,
  patient seated, etc.)

- *palpatory*, manifesting or intensifying through pressure
  applied to a specific area.

Knowing the classification described here is essential for performing
the Test correctly. For this reason, I will give examples to illustrate it.

A *spontaneous* symptom may be a recent ankle sprain, acute
osteoarthritis in any area (wrist, finger, knee etc), a dental abscess,
gastritis, cystitis, a burning sensation from haemorrhoids, a cough or
dysphonia. The organ, the part affected, indicates its malfunction here
and now, and continues to do so. *Spontaneous* pain means that your
ankle hurts even when you do not move it, when you are sitting or
lying down, or when you walk on it. It hurts no matter what.

An example of an *induced kinetic* symptom is so-called tennis elbow,
when the lateral epicondyle hurts *only when* the hand grips the racket
or pours a drink from a bottle, and another is the pain that occurs in
the wrist when spraying window cleaner, or that felt by a motocross
rider when working the accelerator.

An example of an *induced positional* symptom is a stiff neck caused by
a draught of air, occurring when keeping the head turned to the right
(caution: not when turning the head, otherwise it would be *kinetic*!)
or when keeping the head bent forward (but not when bending it!).
Another example is sciatalgia, which occurs only when the patient is
seated, lying prone or on one side. It could be felt in the knee while
crouching or sitting with legs crossed and so on. A combination of
kinetic-positional symptoms is also possible (see Figure 3.2, page 73).

Last, examples of *induced palpatory* symptoms are a sharp pain in
the calf muscle which only occurs when pressure is put on the gluteus
muscles, or stomach pain induced by the patient or the practitioner
putting pressure on the epigastrium with his/her fingers (see Figure
2.11). In such a case, the patient often touches him/herself and
says: 'It hurts (here) when I press here!' Sometimes the two points
coincide, which is the case with many visceral pains. As I have already
mentioned, it goes without saying that not only pain and functional

---

e   In such a case, it can also be defined as *postural*.

impotence may be classified according to this model. A cough may also manifest itself when the patient is lying down or takes a deep breath, and in the same way vertigo can be triggered by moving from a sitting to a lying position. With regard to pain and symptoms which are *not ongoing* at the time of the consultation, if the practitioner cannot perform the Test in his surgery or is unable to visit the patient at home (for example in the case of symptoms experienced at night or during the weekend), it may be possible for the patient to administer the Test him/herself (see section 6.2 in Chapter 6).

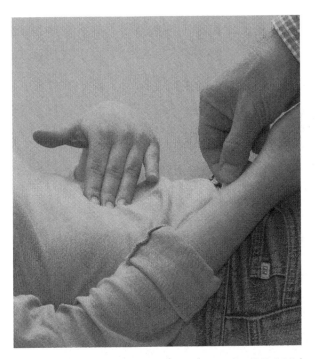

Figure 2.11 The Active Points Test performed on point PC-6 Neiguan for a palpatory symptom (gastric colic and nausea)

2. Explanations and instructions to patient

It will be necessary to explain to the patient exactly what the Active Points Test consists of and give him/her clear instructions, so that the right result is achieved. Simple comprehensible words and sentences should be employed, avoiding the use of medical 'jargon', including that of Chinese medicine, such as *inhibition of neuralgia, myalgia, arthralgia, cortical response, obstruction of the channel, blood stagnation* and so on. I propose a formula which any practitioner can adapt to his or her particular mode of expression:

> 'I will now give you a quick test. Your cooperation is very important, as it will let us know in advance how you will respond to the therapy. Where does it hurt at this moment?'

> The patient will answer: 'It hurts here (touching his shoulder) when I raise my arm to comb my hair.'

> 'Fine, now I'm going to pinch a few points on your skin and you should tell me when I find a point which is *more painful* than the others. Let me know if I cause you too much pain.'

As well as verbal responses, other reactions should also be observed. A complaint, a tightening of the shoulder, a change of expression, a turning-away reflex, movement of the hands or feet, all these will indicate that the bearable pain threshold has been broken. The painful point has therefore been found, but it is not yet an 'active' point. This title will be appropriate only when it has been demonstrated as capable of reducing or neutralising the symptom.

> 'Now close your eyes,[f] while I pinch the point between my fingers, and tell me if the pain I'm causing makes your shoulder pain decrease or disappear. You should also tell me if it doesn't change or if it gets worse. I will try one point at a time (of the painful points found), and out of all the points which improve the symptom, you must tell me which is the most effective.'

It is interesting to note that the most self-confident patients will comment: '*Of course the pain has gone, doctor, because what you are doing hurts more,*' thus stating, without knowing it, Melzack and Wall's gate theory.

---

f   This trick is optional, useful for directing the patient's attention *inwards*.

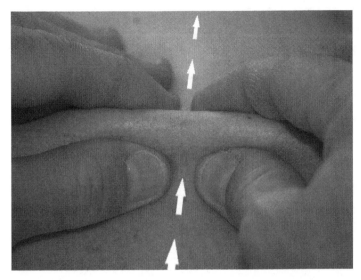

Figure 2.12 Technique of palper rouler *performed on the back with both hands*

3. Looking for the painful points

The points to be tested are the most painful ones inside the chosen area of exploration. They will be identified through meticulously pinching the skin in accordance with the massage technique called *palper rouler* or *pincé roulé,* which mean 'palpating rolling' and 'pinching rolling', and is performed by lifting a fold of skin between the thumb, forefinger and middle finger, first with both hands (Figure 2.12) and then with one. *Once the search is over, the sore point to be tested between thumb and forefinger of one hand must be found* (see examples in Figure 1.1, page 22 and Figure 2.7, page 44). The size of the area where the points are to be found will vary in relation to the extent of the lesion causing the pain or symptom, as this is where it is projected onto the surface of the skin. This is especially true for local points. Small lesions correspond to small areas, large lesions to wide areas. *Information given by the patient is very important.* In fact, the patient will be the one to touch the painful area and indicate a single, precise point, for example on the epicondyle (see Figure 1.2, page 23) or at the centre of the epigastrium (see Figure 2.11, page 49), or more points (internally and in front of the knee joint), or he or she will trace a line, for example along the course of the long head of the biceps, along the sciatic nerve, or he or she will delimit the area, for example on the muscular gluteus or shoulder mass (Figure 2.14). Asking the patient if he can touch the painful area with one finger may narrow down the area to be explored (Figure 2.15).

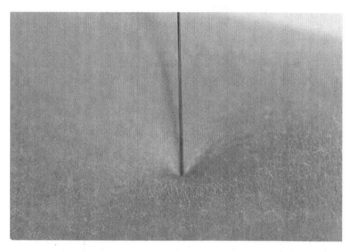

Figure 2.13 The Active Points Test with an acupuncture needle

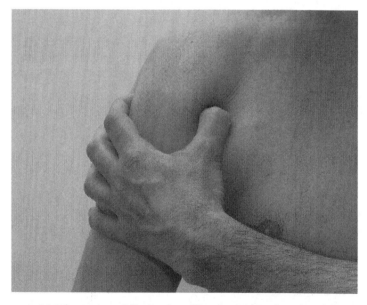

Figure 2.14 The patient delimits the affected area, in this case the muscular mass of the right deltoid

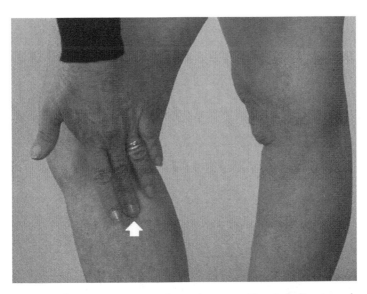

Figure 2.15 The patient narrows down the area affected, indicating where to find the points

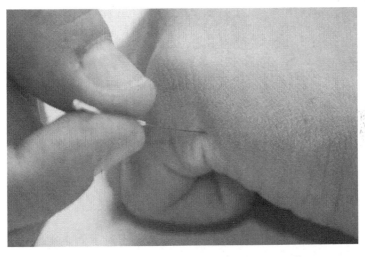

Figure 2.16 The Active Points Test performed with a needle on point SI-3 Houxi Small Intestine

The dimple resulting from the equal distribution of pressure from the needle and the tautness of the skin is evident.

Palpation accompanied by pinching the indicated areas will lead to the identification of some particularly painful points. I say again: even though the patient has been asked to say when *the most painful point* is pinched, it is useful to observe his or her reflexes, any defence muscle contractions or horripilation, as these may happen sooner and have greater significance than words, as well as being an indication that the bearable pain threshold has been broken. We should bear in mind that the individual pain threshold is variable and linked to constitution, upbringing, experience and contingent situations (lack of sleep, physical and psychological stress, menstruation etc.). Having taught dozens of students how to perform the Active Points Test, all I can do is caution readers against using too light or too heavy a hand during the examination. The pinching should start with light pressure, which should be increased gradually until the precise 'dose' for performing the Test is determined. The pain required must be sufficient to neutralise another and no more than that. The cure must not be worse than the disease.

With points having subcutaneous tissue thick or adherent we use the glass stick (see Figure 2.8, page 44) and/or the needle or tip of an empty biro (see Figure 2.9, page 45).

4. Execution of the Test and results

Once the painful points have been identified through the *pincé roulé* method, all that is left is to pinch them using constant pressure and wait for the patient to say what effect each one has on the symptom. A few seconds, ten at most, will be enough. Painful points on areas of taut subcutaneous tissue which have been found by exerting pressure with a glass stick, an empty biro or the auricular massager, will be tested with the same instruments or with a needle. After pinching points on loose skin, if the Test is to be performed with a needle, the tip should be perpendicular to the skin when it makes contact. In this case as well, the patient should be asked to say if the manoeuvre induces any change in his perception of the symptom. The needle should cause a dimple (see Figures 2.9, page 45 and 2.16, page 53), resulting from the equal distribution of pressure exerted by its point and resistance provided by the skin's elasticity. If no such dimple is produced, it is a sign that the pressure being exerted is insufficient or that it has overcome the skin's resistance and the needle has passed through the epidermis. If this occurs, the patient may experience a more intense pain and the manoeuvre will have failed. If the manoeuvre is carried out correctly, the patient should experience a light superficial prick without the slightest discomfort. I recommend taking extra care, especially with those who are new to this method and with patients who are afraid of needles and injections.

Based on the results, the points which improve the symptom will be called *positive* (+) and those that neutralise it will be called *strongly positive* (++). The points which have a small negative effect and those that strongly aggravate the symptom will be called *negative* (−) and *strongly negative* (−−) respectively. Those which fail to change the patient's perception of the symptom will be referred to as *indifferent* (∅).

Classifying the points as *positive, negative* or *indifferent* is indispensable for clinical-statistical verification purposes, and is important for the therapy that will follow the Test. The *positive points* will be used while the *negative* and *indifferent points* will be ruled out. Further details of this will be given later. In terms of their frequency, finding numerous indifferent points is the norm, while, as was predicted by Natour (see page 170), and confirmed later by Romoli,[36] the observation of negative and strongly negative points is very rare both on the soma and on the ear. Positive points, which are essential from the point of view of therapy, are more frequent than negative points but less frequent than indifferent points.

Since it is virtually impossible to remember precisely all the points tested, once the practitioner, especially if he or she is a novice, has removed his hands and looked away from the patient, it is vital that the points be marked, either with a circle (Figure 2.17) or a dot (Figure 3.12, page 99) using a *skin marker*, or by pressing with the nib of an empty biro, even though the mark left by the latter will be short-lived, especially on young patients.

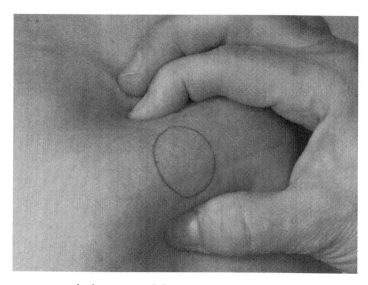

Figure 2.17 Circle drawn round the active point

2.7 THE TEST'S PERSISTENT ACTIVITY EFFECT

Using the Test on a daily basis for over ten years has repeatedly confirmed the observation made in 1994 by my colleagues Mazzanti (personal communication) with regard to somatic acupuncture, and Romoli with regard to auricular puncture.[36] The *persistent activity effect* lies in conserving the therapeutic activity triggered by pinching the point, by pressing with a pen or with the glass stick or through simple contact with a needle. It can vary from a few seconds, which is the amount of time needed to know if the point tested 'works', to a few hours. Sometimes, an improvement in or the disappearance of the symptom are definitive. After noticing a strongly positive point (which neutralises the symptom), and before moving on to explore other points, it is advisable to make sure that the symptom has regained its initial intensity so as to avoid attributing to other points a therapeutic value which they do not really possess.

The *persistent activity effect* has been studied and used brilliantly by Bassani to test classical or auricular points when both the practitioner's hands have been busy with a manoeuvre intended to evaluate the symptom.[37] In these cases, after performing the manoeuvre once, Bassani lightly inserts a needle into the point to be tested and carries out two quick and full rotations, first in a clockwise direction and then anti-clockwise. Immediately afterwards, he repeats the manoeuvre. An example of such a manoeuvre is one for evaluating the strength of the infraspinatus muscle: one hand holds the patient's elbow, with the arm bent at 90° against his or her side, while the other hand provides resistance to a movement intended to over-rotate the arm.

The *persistent activity effect* is essential when the Active Points Test is to be performed in relation to a kinetic symptom on points which are a long way from where it originated. This happens, for example, when a test must be done on a point on the foot for pains in the cervical or dorsal rachis which manifest or are aggravated by walking. Before getting the patient to walk, the chosen point will be stimulated by brief but intense pinching which breaches the pain threshold, or with a needle using Bassani's method.

2.8 SIZE AND ELECTRICAL CHARACTERISTICS OF THE POINTS

It is necessary to mention at this point an important matter in the practice of acupuncture and by extension in the performance of the Test, especially if it is to be carried out with a needle: the size of the points. As reported by Dumitrescu, explorations of the cutis using direct current and alternating current, performed by various researchers, indicated that the average size of Chinese points was between 1 mm² and 1.8 mm².[19] Dumitrescu also conducted a key study in which he analysed with the naked eye and under an optical microscope 10,000 images of points taken from the front (Figure 2.18) and in profile (Figure 2.19) obtained through electronography, which is a technique for recording the emission of electrons from a body onto photosensitive material.

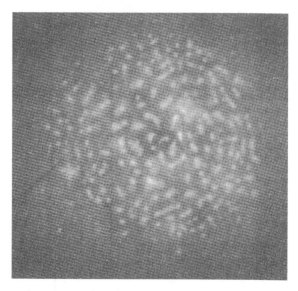

Figure 2.18 Electronography of an acupuncture point (from the front)

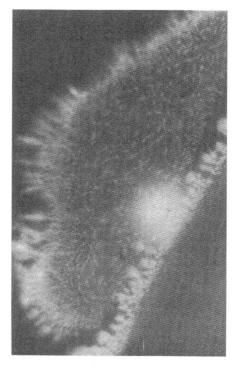

Figure 2.19 Electronography of an acupuncture point (profile)

Electronography has allowed the shape of electrodermal points to be defined and has led to a more precise understanding of their size than exploration with electrodes. Results show that the points are made up of a dark central area which is irregular in shape and has an average diameter of 1.87 mm (with variations from 0.932 mm to 2.66 mm), surrounded by a shiny areola formed by broken concentric lines and with an average diameter of 16.28 mm (with variations from 8.18 mm to 26.20 mm). We are faced with an extremely small area, a target into which acupuncture needles, with a diameter of between 0.20 mm and 0.40 mm, barely fit. This is another valid reason for choosing to pinch the skin rather than stimulate it with a needle, or at least to do this first. Furthermore, as anatomical reference points can vary individually, it is suggested that newcomers who want to use a needle during the Test look for points electronically so that the Test will be more effective. Only an accurate study of the position of the points and clinical experience will make the use of a pointscope unnecessary.

It was Di Stanislao (see pages 160–163), who observed the link between electrical changes and the activity of points. The author detected a constant relation between the positive reaction of points to the Test and a decrease in resistance to electrical current passing over these areas, and between negative reactions and an increase in electrical resistance. This should not be interpreted as meaning that every point showing a change in resistance to the passage of electrical current must necessarily correspond to a positive or negative point. Nevertheless, this observation makes us think about how a *clinical sign*, in this case the patient's positive or negative response to superficial stimulation with a needle, can often be measured, if one has the right technology.

While looking for points using electronic technology, I have personally been able to confirm Dumitrescu's observation about two phenomena which concern them, although I have not correlated activity and electrical change: the *dilation of the point's area* and *multiplication*. The first is an enlargement of the low resistance area to a few centimetres, while the second is an increase in the number of points. Dumitrescu called these changes *fenestration occlusion*. As my priority was to try to confirm my observation and to perfect the Test, I did not explore the points systematically as Di Stanislao and Romoli did before testing them with a needle, since I did not have at my disposal the equipment necessary for evaluating the smallest variations in resistance.

Although haste is the enemy of a good diagnosis and of the right therapy, an investigation should not be overly long, so as to avoid exhausting both the patient and the practitioner. To compensate for the inconvenience, manual techniques can be used in order to look for points: using the tip of the forefinger to look for the point at the centre of the dimple described by classical authors, particularly Soulié de Morant,[38] or lightly prodding the small area of the point so as to find the most sensitive part which would correspond to the acupuncture point. In actual fact, the area which is most sensitive to pain is the part surrounding the real point, which most authors consider insensitive. The discovery of a hyperalgesic zone, however, indicates the close proximity of the point.

2.9 DISTANCE BETWEEN THE POINTS

After 1929 the People's Republic of China officially adopted the decimal metric system. The modern (shì) cùn 市寸 is equal to ⅓ of a decimetre, and its decimal submultiple is the fēn 市分. Traditional Chinese Medicine (TCM) uses the antique Cùn 寸 (pronounced tsun), or 'distance', as its unit of measurement. It is an 'individual' segment corresponding to the distance between the proximal interphalangeal joint and the distal interphalangeal joint of the middle finger, or rather the maximum width of the thumb at the distal interphalangeal joint (Figure 2.20) All distances between one acupuncture point and another, and between one point and its specific anatomical reference, are multiples of the cùn, as shown in those pictures which contain a ruler (see Figure 2.2, page 37). The measurement of the distance between the points is important where there is no clear reference, such as on the sides, the back and the central areas of the arm, the forearm, thigh and leg. As seen in the previous paragraph, localising the point can present difficulties, especially for beginners, so it is a good rule to use a stick that is the length of the patient's cùn or a point protractor (Figure 2.21), at least in the beginning.

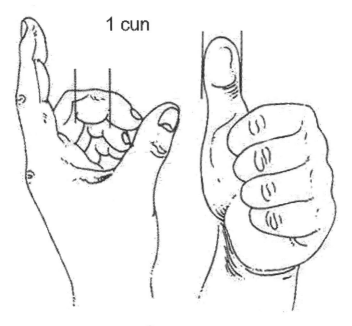

Figure 2.20 Acupuncture unit of measurement

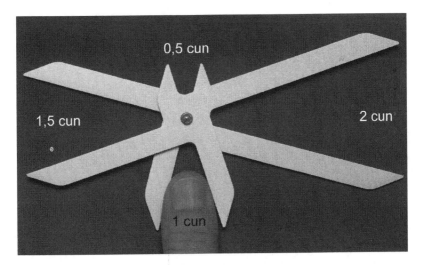

Figure 2.21 Cunmeter

2.10 CLINICAL-STATISTICAL OBSERVATION EVIDENCE

Any rational spirit, when faced with claims about the discovery of new phenomena capable of changing current opinion in a given field of knowledge, will require evidence as to its truth and repeatability. In this paragraph, I will report the data from my clinical study concluded in 1995, which is still valid today.

As I have already explained, the Active Points Test makes it possible to find out in advance of therapy if the cutaneous points belonging to classical acupuncture, auricular puncture and other reflex therapy maps are really effective. The patient is an invaluable source of information in terms of the therapeutic regulation of his internal cybernetic circuit: *symptom* → *stimulation* → *change in symptom*. It is based on the observation of a phenomenon which I have called *latent awareness of the active point*, which means that a patient with an ongoing, continuous and clearly perceived symptom, through palpation or simple contact without penetration by the tip of a needle on cutaneous points, can be made aware of their therapeutic capacity and so pass on an immediate (generally from 2–5 seconds) improvement, neutralisation or deterioration in the symptom.

After observing the phenomenon for the first time, I devoted myself researching it systematically using a sample of 260 patients, of whom 156 were female F (60%) and 104 were male M (40%), with an average age of about 42. Ongoing symptoms at the time of the consultation were subdivided according to system:

Locomotive system, 144 cases (74F and 70M), 55.38%

- 29 cases of cervicalgia
- 9 cases of cervicobrachialgia (of which 2 were of brachialgia only)
- 27 cases of shoulder pain
- 12 cases of epicondylalgia
- 2 cases of medial epicondylitis
- 3 cases of wrist pain
- 4 cases of chiralgia (1 carpal tunnel syndrome, 1 painful trigger finger and 2 rizarthrosis of the thumb)
- 1 case of phantom arm pain

- 1 case of intercostal pain
- 7 cases of back pain
- 10 cases of lumbalgia
- 24 cases of lumbosciatalgia
- 1 case of coccydynia
- 4 cases of coxalgia
- 2 cases of gonalgia
- 3 cases of foot pain (1 of Morton's neuroma)
- 5 cases of localised myalgia

Digestive and chewing system, 32 cases (19 F and 13M), 12.31%

- 17 cases of gastralgia
- 2 cases of dysphagia
- 8 cases of chronic abdominal pain
- 1 case of anal pain
- 1 case of temporomandibular joint pain
- 2 cases of odontalgia
- 1 case of burning mouth syndrome

Ear, nose and throat and respiratory system,
32 cases (19F and 13M), 12.31%

- 3 cases of pharyngodynia
- 14 cases of nasal occlusion
- 2 cases of otalgia
- 2 cases of paranasal sinus pain (Figure 2.22)
- 2 cases of dyspnoea
- 3 cases of coughing
- 4 cases of tinnitus
- 2 cases of vertigo

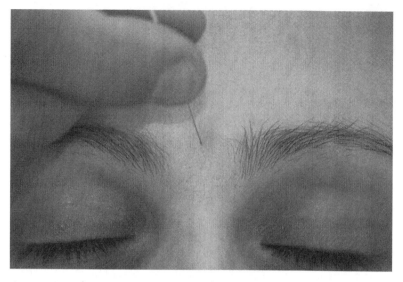

Figure 2.22 The Active Points Test with acupuncture needle on extra point Yintang for a frontal headache caused by sinusitis

Cardiovascular system, 2 cases (2F), 0.77%

- 1 case of tachycardia
- 1 case of periphlebitis

Neuropsychological and sensory system, 40 cases (33F and 7M), 15.38%

- 1 case of localised paresthesia
- 1 case of lower limb palsy
- 23 cases of headache
- 7 cases of neuralgia (4 of trigeminal neuralgia, 1 pectoral neuralgia caused by influenza, 1 herpetic, 1 facial *a frigore*)
- 1 case of pectoral neuralgia
- 1 case of anosmia
- 1 case of insomnia
- 3 cases of psychomotor agitation

- 1 case of intention tremor

- 1 case of depression

Various systems, 10 cases (9F and 1M), 3.85%

- 5 cases of pruritus

- 4 cases of burning/stinging sensation (2 vaginal, 2 of the eyelid)

- 1 case of dysmenorrhea

The type of symptom was *spontaneous* (always present during the execution of the Test) in 229 cases out of 260, equal to 88.08%, and *induced* in 31 cases, equal to 11.92%, divided as follows:

- *kinetic* (present only during the execution of certain movements) in 16 cases, equal to 6.15%

- *positional* (present only when assuming certain positions) in 10 cases, equal to 3.85%

- *palpatory* (present only during palpation) in 5 cases, equal to 1.92%.

As for the duration of the symptom, taking into account how some patients may tend to exaggerate the duration of their problems due to lack of memory, the result was an average of about 16½ months (with 1 month equal to 30 days), with a minimum period of 1 day and a maximum of 50 years.

The distribution of results is as follows:

< 1 week	26 cases, equal to 10%
≥ 1 week and < 1 month	54 cases, equal to 20.77%
≥ 1 month and < 6 months	95 cases, equal to 36.54%
≥ 6 months and < 2 years	42 cases, equal to 16.15%
≥ 2 years and < 10 years	30 cases, equal to 11.54%
≥ 10 years	13 cases, equal to 5%

For 141 patients out of 260 (54.23%), the Test was carried out only on classical points (PC). For 25 patients (9.62%), it was only performed on auricular points (PA), while for 94 patients (36.15%), it was executed on both types of points. Overall, classical points were tested in relation to 235 patients (90.38%) and auricular points in relation to 119 (45.77%).

For the 235 patients in relation to whom classical points were tested, the following was found:

- In 41 cases: only positive points (+), equal to 17.45%

- In 89 cases: only strongly positive points (++), equal to 37.87%

- In 75 cases: positive and strongly positive point (+, ++), equal to 31.91%

- In 11 cases: positive, strongly positive and negative points (+, ++, −), equal to 4.68%

- In 3 cases: positive, strongly positive, negative and strongly negative points (+, ++, −, −−), equal to 1.28%

- In 5 cases: positive and negative points (+, −), equal to 2.13%

- In 1 case: strongly positive and negative points (++, −), equal to 0.43%.

In 1 case only, negative and strongly negative points (−, −−) alone were noticed, equal to 0.43%. Finally, in 9 cases there was absolutely no response from points to the Test: these are the *absolute non-responders*, 3.83%.

Positive points (+ and ++) were found among the *classical points* in 225 cases, with a frequency of 95.74%, while overall, negative points (− and −−) were found in 21 cases, with a frequency of 8.94%.

For the 119 patients in relation to whom *auricular points* were tested, the following was found:

- In 35 cases: only positive points (+), equal to 29.41%

- In 69 cases: only strongly positive points (++), equal to 57.98%

- In 9 cases: positive and strongly positive points (+, ++), equal to 7.56%.

In one case only (here as well) negative and strongly negative points (−, −−) alone were noticed, equal to 0.84%, which also corresponds to the overall frequency of negative points.

Lastly, in 5 cases (all belonging to the 9 mentioned above) there was no response at all to the Test: *absolute non-responders*, 4.20%

Of the 260 patients, 238 were treated (91.54%); 22 cases were not treated, of which: 6 were from the 9 *absolute non-responders*, 1 gave up for financial reasons, 1 due to an unpleasant effect caused by the Test (an after-effect of puncture in a patient suffering from multiple sclerosis), another 2 because they suffered from needle phobia and, lastly, 11 were cases in which the Test was performed as a demonstration during conferences and seminars to present the methodology. These 11 patients did, however, receive an acupuncture session after the Test, but the results were not checked directly by the author. Of the 9 patients classed as *absolute non-responders*, 2 were treated by acupuncture alone, without appreciable results.

From the body of data reported above, it can be deduced that:

> *The Active Points Test confirms the therapeutic activity (positive +, and strongly positive ++) of classical acupuncture and auricular puncture points in 250 cases out of 260, equal to 96.15%, which statistically is very reliable.*

The overall number of sessions in which the treated patients took part was 660, with an average of 2.77 sessions per patient, varying from a minimum of 1 session only to a maximum of 11, divided as follows:

- In 82 cases: 1 session, equal to 34.45%

- In 56 cases: 2 sessions, equal to 23.53%

- In 37 cases: 3 sessions, equal to 15.55%

- In 22 cases: 4 sessions, equal to 9.24%

- In 17 cases: 5 sessions, equal to 7.14%

- In 11 cases: 6 sessions, equal to 4.62%

- In 6 cases: 7 sessions, equal to 2.25%

- In 3 cases: 8 sessions, equal to 1.26%

- In 2 cases: 9 sessions, equal to 0.84%

- In 1 case: 10 sessions, equal to 0.42%

- In 1 case: 11 sessions, equal to 0.42%.

Of the 238 patients treated:

- 214 received only acupuncture/auricular puncture (AP), equal to 89.92%

- 17 received acupuncture/auricular puncture and mesotherapy (MT), equal to 7.14%

- 2 received acupuncture/auricular puncture and moxibustion, equal to 0.84%

- 1 received AP, MT and electroacupuncture (EAP), equal to 0.42%

- 1 received AP, MT and vetebral manipulation (MV), equal to 0.42%

- 1 received AP, MV and cortisonic therapy by mouth, equal to 0.42%

- 1 received AP, MT, neural therapy (NE) and the application of magnets to acupunture points (AM), equal to 0.42%

- 1 received AP, MT and Carbamazepina, equal to 0.42%.

Only the points which resulted *positive* (+) and *strongly positive* (++) were treated; the *negative* (−) and *strongly negative* (−−) points were excluded from the therapy so as not to complicate the analysis of data relating to it. Treatment was interrupted when no improvement (even minimal) was seen for 2 consecutive sessions and in every case where there was complete remission of the symptom. The evaluation of the results was made by asking the patient, at the first consultation and at the beginning of every session, to express as a percentage between 0% (no symptom) and 100% (maximum intensity of symptom) the 'amount' of the symptom, after agreeing to attribute the value of 100% to the symptom as it presented at the first visit. The results of therapy were as follows:

- good in 154 cases, 64.71%

- moderate in 33 cases, 13.87%

- insufficient in 16 cases, 6.72%

- none in 10 cases, 4.20%.[g]

Furthermore:

- moderate with AP, good with MT in 1 case, 0.42%

- moderate with AP, good with MT and MV in 1 case 0.42%

- moderate with AP, good with AP and Moxa in 1 case, 0.42%

- insufficient with AP, good with MT in 8 cases, 3.36%

- insufficient with AP, good with MT and Carbamazepina in 1 case, 0.42%

- insufficient with AP, good with MV and cortisonic by mouth in 1 case, 0.42%

- none with AP, good with MT in 1 case, 0.42%

- insufficient with AP, moderate with MT in 1 case, 0.42%

- moderate with AP and Moxa in 1 case, 0.42%

- none with AP, moderate with MT in 1 case, 0.42%

- insufficient with AP and MT, moderate with NE and AM in 1 case, 0.42%

- insufficient with both AP and MT in 3 cases, 1.26%

- none with AP, MT and EAP in 1 case, 0.42%.

2.11 NON-RESPONDERS

Cases in which the Test fails to register the presence of the active points are called *absolute non-responders*. Those in which the Test indicates that the points explored have some therapeutic capacity, but in which therapy does not alter the symptom have been named *relative non-responders* by Romoli. I nevertheless treated 2 of the 9 *absolute non-responders* with acupuncture and, where this was insufficient, I added mesotherapy and in one case electroacupuncture as well. The Test's

---

g   *Key:* good: complete remission of symptom or above or equal to 75%
     moderate: remission below 75% but above or equal to 50%
     insufficient: remission below 50%
     none: no or negligible remission

failure to register the presence of the active points may suggest that therapy on cutaneous points is not indicated. Like Di Stanislao, I tested points belonging to other reflex therapy maps (the skull, the hand, the foot, the nose and the oral mucosa) on a small number of patients and verified that the Test is also effective on points other than those of classical acupuncture and auricular puncture.

Chapter 3

CHOOSING POINTS

3.1 TWO CRITERIA FOR CHOOSING

Just as blood and urine analyses can be requested by any doctor irrespective of his specialisation, so the Active Points Test may be performed by any therapist who treats 'through' the skin. The type and number of analyses ordered will depend on the experience of the doctor, as well as on the patient's symptoms. Any doctor may request 'routine tests': blood count, complete urine etc., and every specialist has his own 'specific protocol': hormones, enzymes, peptides, electrolytes etc. In the same way, the type and number of points to be subjected to the Active Points Test will vary depending on the training and experience of the practitioner. It goes without saying that an experienced traditional acupuncturist, after examining the pulse and the tongue, will have in mind some points for treating the onset of the disease and some for treating its root cause. An inexperienced physiotherapist, shiatsu or tuina practitioner, or mesotherapist will instinctively concentrate on the two or three points indicated by the patient.

Nevertheless, since the words 'villa', 'castle' and 'tower' cannot be understood if the term 'house' is not recognised, I suggest two criteria for choosing the points, which will allow anyone to set up the Active Points Test in a way that best suits his or her training and – why not? – intuition.

3.2 QUICK CHOICE POINTS

These are the easiest, most obvious points. The amount of time needed to identify them is short or very short, in terms of *speed of decision, intuition* and *judgement*. Local, paravertebral and spondyloid points are part of this group. More than one point from each of these groups may be found, especially in relation to chronic, prolonged illnesses, and the most painful ones should be selected for carrying out the Test. The choice of these points is based on a clinical and neurological knowledge of western medicine, even though they often correspond exactly to acupuncture points.

1. Local points

Local points are found on the skin over the symptom site (Figures 3.1, 3.2 and 3.3). This is the point that troubles the patient, that hurts continuously or when he or she moves, assumes a certain position, coughs etc. In relation to epicondylitis pains, the local point is on the elbow. It is found on the shoulder for periarthritis, on the sternum or the back for a cough, 'above' the stomach for heartburn and so on. For an acupuncturist, local points often coincide with traditional 'local points'. This is also true for mesotherapists and practitioners of connective tissue massage, even though they may not know the Chinese terms. Local points are undeniably those which are less likely to require practitioners to have specialist knowledge of anatomy and acupuncture channels. It is worth bearing in mind that no lay person, no matter how *latently aware they are of the active point*, would dream of massaging themselves at point ST-38 Tiaokou for shoulder pain, that no one would ever think of using a finger to put pressure on the space between the second and third toe, on point ST-44 Neiting, to alleviate toothache or stomach ache. The reason is that these points are simply too far away, physically and conceptually, from the seat of the symptom. However, those who have studied the odd acupuncture textbook are aware that the effectiveness of the two points on those symptoms is widely known and probable. But that is the point – they must have studied it.

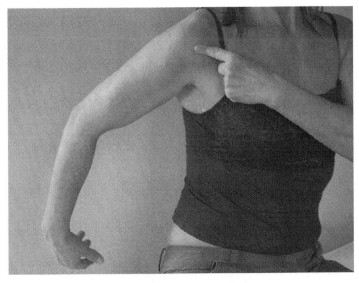

Figure 3.1 Local point indicated by patient suffering from tendonitis in the long head of the biceps

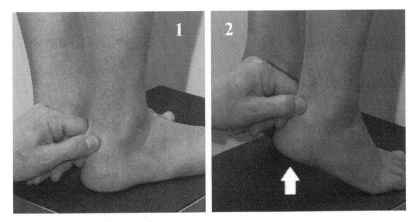

Figure 3.2 Local point for inflammation of the Achilles tendon, with kinetic pain manifesting when standing on tiptoes

(1) Identification of most painful point. (2) Execution of Test during the movement.

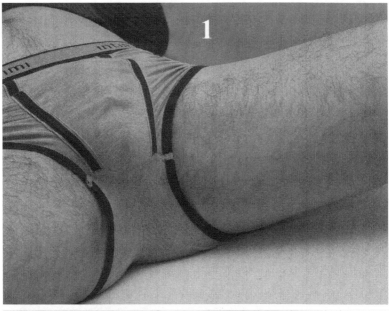

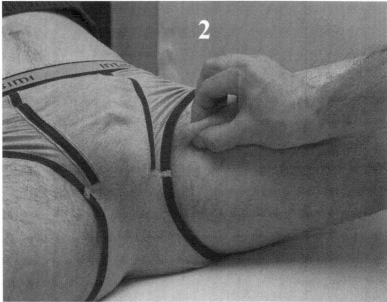

Figure 3.3 (1) Kinetic-positional symptom (left groin pain which manifests while running and when supine with legs apart) (2) Test of local point on skin projection of pubic insertion of adductor muscles

The tongue ever turns to the aching tooth: Nature makes us touch the spot that hurts with our hand. The more focalised the injury causing the symptom, the fewer painful points will be found by pinching the skin, down to a single point only.

2. Paravertebral points

In addition to the local point or points, there are the *paravertebral points* (Figures 3.4, 3.5 and 3.7) They are found along the lines that run parallel to the two sides of the vertebral column, 2–3 cm (the width of two fingers, or 1.5 cun) from the spinal apophysis of the vertebrae. Choosing paravertebral points is quick, provided that a map of dermatomes is available (Figure 3.7). A *dermatome* or *segmental field*, as it was called by Sherrington,[39,40] who was the first person to define it electrically, is the area of skin innervated by a spinal nerve. Dermatome C7 is the sensory field of the seventh cervical nerve, dermatome L2 is that of the second lumbar nerve and so on. In a case of epicondylitis, the most painful local point (above and around the epicondyle) and the most painful paraverterbral point of dermatomes C5, C6 and C7 (Figure 3.6) will be located and tested. Due to individual anatomical variations, it is a good idea to explore the dermatomes above and below as well. The paravertebral cutis is suitable for use in learning the *pincé roulé* (Figure 3.5), the massage technique used for locating the painful points which will be subjected to the Active Points Test.

> The *posterior* or *dorsal* branches of the spinal nerves stimulate the muscles into movement and supply nerves to the skin in the dorsal area of the torso; they are arranged in a regular manner and have common features. The posterior branches are generally smaller than the corresponding anterior branches, with the exception of the first two cervical dorsal branches. After leaving the nerve, the posterior branches cross the space which separates the transverse processes of two adjoining vertebrae and reach the muscles of the vertebral recesses which are innervated by two branches, the *medial* and the *lateral*. One of the two branches also stretches to the skin above.[41]

The paravertebral points correspond anatomically to the emergence of the posterior branch of the spinal nerve at the point where it separates into the lateral and medial branches (Figures 3.5, 3.6 and 3.7), and coincide with the transporting-shu points on the Urinary Bladder Channel. 'Local points' are also relevant to symptoms relating to the vertebral column (cervicalgia, dorsalgia, lumbalgia). I believe I have already explained the reasons why I was persuaded to include them among the quick choice points.

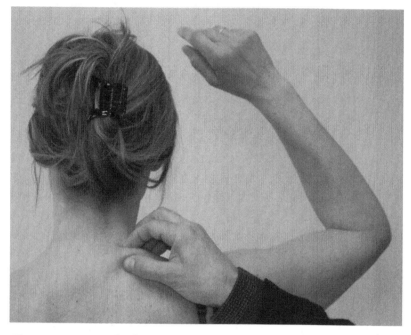

Figure 3.4 Paravertebral point, tested in relation to kinetic pain in the elbow which manifests while raising the arm (see Figure 1.2)

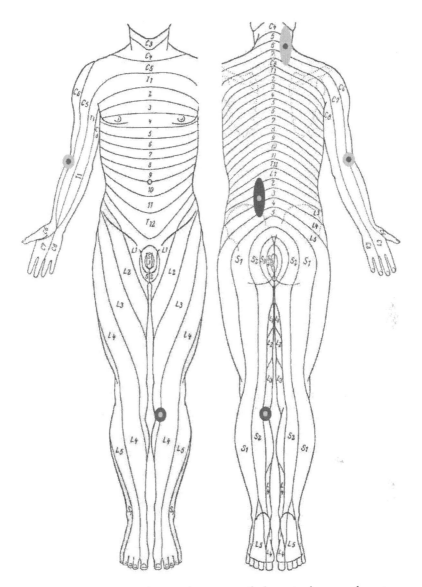

Figure 3.5 Anterior and posterior maps of the spinal nerve dermatomes showing the areas to explore in order to identify local and paravertebral points (C5-C7 and L2-L4) for left knee pain and epicondylitis in the right arm
The internal circles represent the most painful points, which are to be subjected to the Test.

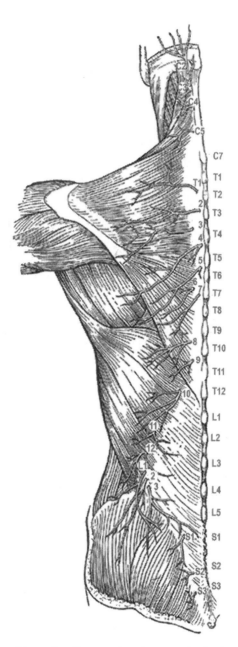

Figure 3.6 Lateral branches (innervating the paravertebral points) and medial branches (innervating the spondyloid points) of the posterior branches of the spinal nerves

(See Balboni *et al.*, note 41.)

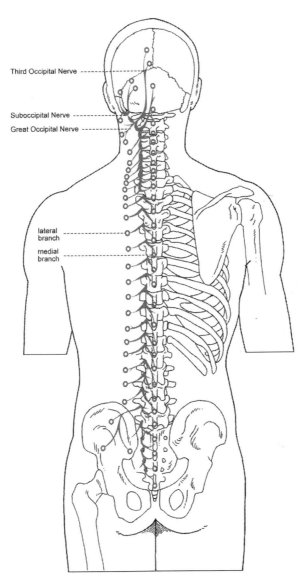

Figure 3.7 Lateral branches (paravertebral points) and medial branches (spondyloid points) of the posterior branches of the spinal nerves

It is interesting to note the link between the lateral branches and the acupuncture back points on the Bladder Channel (transporting-shu), and between the medial branches and the points on the Governing Vessel. The bifurcation of the posterior branches into medial and lateral branches coincides with the Huatuojiaji extraordinary points (see Balboni *et al.*, note 41).

3. Spondyloid points

The spondyloid points are optional and complementary to the paravertebral points, and will be located on the posterior or spondyloid sagittal plane, which touches all the spinal processes (the protuberances) of the vertebrae, from the first cervical vertebra to the coccyx, and is served by the medial branch of the posterior nerve branch (Figures 3.5, 3.6 and 3.7). A dermatome map will be used to locate these points. In diseases of the vertebral column, spondyloid points may coincide with local points.

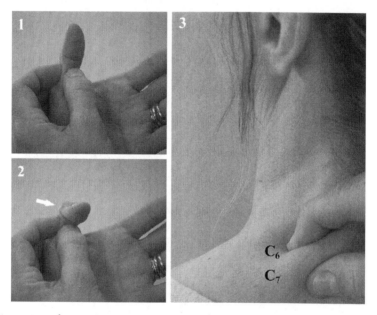

Figure 3.8 The Active Points Test in accordance with the quick choice criterion for a kinetic symptom: pain in the distal interphalangeal joint of the thumb, manifesting during flexion

(1) and (2) Pinching the most painful local point. (3) Pinching the paravertebral point at the level of C6-C7, on the same dermatome to which the anatomical seat of the symptom belongs, while the patient flexes her thumb.

Local points, paravertebral and spondyloid points constitute the Active Points Test protocol for my students of mesotherapy, acupuncture and medical reflexology, and for the courses in shiatsu, physiotherapy and Traditional Chinese Medicine (TCM) to which I am invited to demonstrate the Test. Figures 3.8 and 3.9 show two examples of a sequence of movements for executing the Test in accordance with the quick choice criteria, with the exclusion of the spondyloid points.

For practitioners of reflex therapies like auricular puncture, cranial puncture, nose and facial puncture, hand and foot puncture, and puncture of the oral mucosa,[42] the quick choice points are those that have the closest somatotopic relationship to the symptom, reported in the relevant reference books (e.g. cough = lungs, lumbalgia = lumbar vertebrae, etc.).

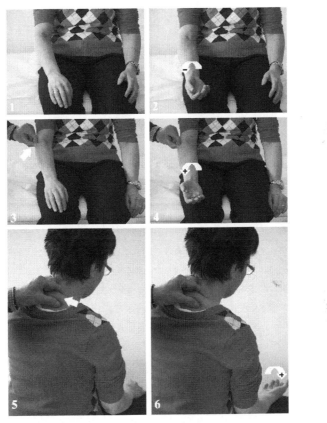

Figure 3.9 The Active Points Test used in accordance with the quick choice criterion in relation to kinetic pain in the right elbow (from epicondylitis) which manifests when during supination of the hand

(1) At rest. (2) Painful supination of the hand (−). (3) Identifying the painful local point (arrow on elbow). (4) Test on local point: painless supination (+). (5) Identifying the painful paravertebral point (arrow on neck). (6) Test on paravertebral point: painless supination (+).

3.3 REASONED CHOICE POINTS

These are points chosen on the basis of a detailed (but not necessarily slow) diagnostic reasoning. They are not in contrast with the quick choice points, and one criterion does not exclude the other. More space will be given to techniques based on the principles of TCM because they are more widespread. Other techniques will be described briefly and a few general pointers will be given. Until there is irrefutable proof of the existence of the Qi and the Channels, it is possible that the use of distal points in therapies of western origin will be considered 'irrational'. However, since the Active Points Test clearly works on its own even on points inferred from acupuncture maps – better still it often reveals these points to be the most powerful in terms of therapeutic activity – even a western practitioner may feel completely justified in using it. The following paragraphs examine how the reasoned choice points are selected in accordance with the different methodologies.

3.4 TRADITIONAL CHINESE ACUPUNCTURE, TUINA AND SHIATSU

In both classical and modern textbooks, points are organised into formulas or combinations. When it is possible to find the exact seat of a symptom, such as a burning sensation in the lower abdomen when urinating, local and distal points are prescribed. The need to make a distinction does not arise when faced with a symptom which is not easily localised, such as tiredness or dizziness, or pain which spreads or moves around the abdomen. Tradition invests the distal points with greater therapeutical power, although the high number of extra points makes us think otherwise. I have randomly taken from contemporary authors a few formulas with a low number of points.

Stiff neck[43]
Main points: Laozhenxue (Extra), Xuanzhong (GB-39), Houxi (SI-3), Ahshi points, Yanglao (SI-6).

All the points are treated on the side affected. Usually, Laozhenxue (Extra), Xuanzhong (GB-39) or Yanglao (SI-6) are manipulated with moderate or strong force initially. As the needle is being rotated, the patient is asked to rotate his or her head.[h]

Supplementary points:

Headache: Fengchi GB-20, Waiguan TE-5.

Shoulder and back pain: Quyuan SI-13, Dazhu BL-11, Janwaishu SI-14.

Inability to lift or lower the head: Lieque LU-7, or Dazhu BL-11 and Jinggu BL-64.

Inability to look backwards: Zhizheng SI-17, Janwaishu SI-14.

Rectal prolapse and haemorrhoids[44]

The main local point is GV-1, needle inserted at right angles. If necessary the needle may be directed to the right or to the left so that the feeling of penetration radiates outwards into the anus. Subsidiary local points like BL-30, BL-32, BL-35 and BL 54 may also be used. The main distal point is BL-57 to be used for dispersion.

Variations:

PC-8 dispersion for heat signs.

SP-10 dispersion for bleeding caused by heat.

BL-25, ST-37 dispersion for constipation.

GV-20 moxa for haemorrhoids or rectal prolapse due to Qi Sinking, the moxa stick may be used for 15 minutes.

CV-8 moxa for Qi Sinking, moxa cones on ginger slices and on salt.

Ankle[16]

Ankle pain is usually caused by an invasion of cold and damp and from a local stagnation of the Qi due to excessive use of the joint. The main points to use are:

SP-5 Shangqiu is one of the two most important points (together with GB-40 Qiuxu). As well as being a local point, it eliminates damp and, since it is the *jing* point, it acts on the joints. It is usually

---

h   Here too, the patient is instructed to move the neck during manipulation.

punctured in combination with GB-40 Qiuxu. GB-40 Qiuxu is used if the pain is in the external part of the ankle, and is often penetrated using a heated needle.

ST-41 Jiexi is used when the pain is in the neck of the foot. It also eliminates damp. It should be punctured at right angles,[i] to a depth of at least 1.25 cm.

It follows from this that, for traditional acupuncturists, the Active Points Test can act as a guide for choosing between a few select points, or for checking whether the hypothetical active point diagnosis for a given symptom is correct and, if it is not, for directing the search elsewhere. In the example above taken from Ross regarding haemorrhoids, distal point BL-57 Chengshan (see Figure 3.10) and all supplementary points indicated for the patient's feelings of heaviness and burning could be tested first by pinching and then with a needle, before insertion. The same reasoning can be applied to shiatsu and again to tuina, the practice of which is founded on the same theoretical assumptions as traditional acupuncture. There now follow a few suggestions for practitioners of TCM who want to put the Active Points Test into practice. Points chosen which are not located on the median lines may be tested on both sides of the body, first on the right and then on the left, since different responses may result depending on which side is punctured. This observation is reported in ancient and modern treatises and is well known to practitioners of traditional acupuncture. One example from among many is the puncturing of ST-38 to treat the homolateral and contralateral shoulder.[46,47] In relation to the Test, it often happens that the same point, even an extra point, is positive on one side and indifferent on the other. In rarer cases, the effect is the opposite. In terms of electric resistance, the same phenomenon was observed by Dumitrescu and his colleagues.[19] Knowledge of the course of the Main and Collateral Channels, the Muscle Regions and the Extraordinary Channels, as well as the correlation between the sensory organs and the endocrine and metabolic organs, are the foundation of a sensible choice. For *Bi* syndrome in the shoulder, it is essential to know which channels are assigned to the movements limited by the disease. In a

---

i   Why is the patient not expected to move the part affected during needle manipulation for problems with the ankle, knee, hip and fingers as well?

case of perverse energy or internal imbalance syndrome relating to the throat it is essential to know that the fauces are controlled by the Lung, Spleen and Liver Channels, and in the area of the ear energy from the Kidneys, Gall Bladder and Small Intestine is expressed, and so on.

The Test will concentrate at first on the key points of the Extraordinary Channels, because here the Qi's circulation is not seasonal, but has a relatively constant flow. Their energetic 'pressure' depends on the mutual balance and energy of the Main Channels connected to them (*Yang* and *Yin* groups of the upper and lower limbs), and whose flow is subject to seasonal rhythms and to daily and hourly tides. Once the strategic points of the Extraordinary Channels have been tested, the Test will move on to those of the Main Channels. Meticulous palpation of the entire course of the channels using the *pincé roulé* and biro methods will lead to the identification of areas of painful cellulite to be tested, even if they do not correspond perfectly to traditional points (Figure 3.10).

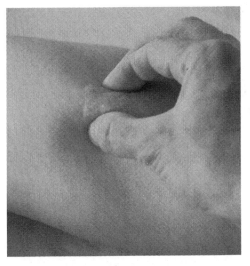

Figure 3.10 The Active Points Test in accordance with the quick choice criterion, for burning from haemorrhoids, performed on the most painful point in the area of the BL-57 Chengshan Urinary Bladder, asking the patient to communicate any variations in perception of the symptom
The infiltration of cellulite in the area of skin pinched is noticeable.

There now follows a brief description of the Extraordinary Channels and of the 'functional' groups of points on both the Extraordinary and the Main Channels, with related lists. The extra points have been missed out due to lack of space. The functional groups of points are arranged in order of the priority that I have attributed to them with respect to the Active Points Test. It goes without saying that any practitioner may change this in accordance with his or her own reasoning. For further details of TCM, the reader is referred to the specified texts and atlases listed in the endnotes section.[7,14,15,16,17,31,43,45]

The Extraordinary Channels

With the exception of the *Dumai* and the *Renmai*, the Extraordinary Channels 'borrow' points from the Main Channels. *Dumai* and *Renmai* have a collateral (Luo) channel and Luo points.

Dumai 'Governing Vessel': this is the *Yang* channel which rises up along the posterior median sagittal plane, harvesting and balancing the *Yang* energy of the upper and lower limb. Its points are tested in relation to symptoms concerning the vertebral column and the musculoskeletal system, as well as for visceral diseases, since it acts as a relay to the spinal cord. Testing the points of the 'Governing Vessel' is also useful for ailments relating to the head and for mental disorders.

Renmai 'Conception Vessel': this is the *Yin* channel which rises up along the anterior median sagittal plane, harvesting and balancing the *Yin* energy of the lower and upper limb. It is important to test its points in relation to all symptoms concerning visceral diseases in the organs situated along the median plane: mouth and incisors, tongue, larynx, trachea, oesophagus, bronchial tube, stomach, duodenum, pancreas, transverse colon, small intestine, bladder, uterus, vagina, prostate and penis. The Front-Mu points, otherwise known as 'herald', are found on the *Renmai* channel and are to be tested immediately or as a second option.

Chongmai 'Thoroughfare Vessel': *Yin* in nature, it is also known by the name *vital vessel* or *defence vessel* and runs inside the body on the median plane, uniting the *Yin* energy of the Conception Vessel and the *Yang* energy of the Governing Vessel. It also has a small surface area which borrows some points from the Kidney Channel. Its points should be tested for symptoms relating to visceral diseases, for all types of abdominal colic, metabolic disorders, and problems relating to the urinary passage and the menstrual cycle.

Daimai 'Girdle Vessel': this channel is *Yang* in nature and harvests the energy of the Gall Bladder Channel, condensing it, as the name implies, into the form of a girdle. Its points should be tested for all diseases of the pelvis, the liver and the gall bladder.

Yangweimai 'Yang Link Vessel': is also known as the *Yang Regulator Vessel*, and links the *Yang* channels of the lower part of the body to those of the upper part and to the Governing Vessel. Its points are to be tested for ailments of the thorax and for those in the shoulder and head area.

Yinweimai 'Yin Link Vessel': it is also known as the *Yin Regulator Vessel*, and links the *Yin* channels of the lower part of the body to the Conception Vessel. As for the previous channels, its points are to be tested for ailments of the thorax and for those in the shoulder and head area.

Yangqiaomai 'Yang Heel Vessel': it also takes the name *Yang Motility Vessel*, and connects low *Yang* energy to high *Yang* energy. Its points should be tested for articular symptoms relating to the lower limbs and the shoulder, and for diseases of the head.

Yinqiaomai 'Yin Heel Vessel': it also takes the name *Yin Motility Vessel*, and connects low *Yin* energy to high *Yin* energy. As for the previous vessel, its points should be tested for articular symptoms relating to the lower limbs and the shoulder, and for diseases of the head.

Functional groups of acupuncture points

The eight *confluent* or *opening points* (*key-opening* points for French authors) of the Extraordinary Channels are to be given absolute priority when performing the Active Points Test in accordance with the quick choice criterion for any symptom, since the imbalance in the Main Channels *always* manifests on the flow of the Extraordinary Channels. The *Yang* channels (*Dumai, Daimai, Yangqiaomai, Yangweimai*) give information about the energy of the *Yang* Main Channels (Large Intestine, Stomach, Small Intestine, Bladder, Triple Heater and Gall Bladder). Likewise, the *Yin* channels (*Renmai, Chongmai, Yinqiaomai,*

Yinweimai) give information about the Main Channels of the same nature (Lung, Spleen, Heart, Kidney, Pericardium and Liver). The opening points, on the Main Channels, 'open' the Extraordinary Channels, allowing the former to pour out part of their energy when *full* or to recharge themselves when *empty*.

TABLE 3.1 THE 8 CONFLUENT POINTS

	Yang		*Yin*	
Hand	*Dumai* SI-3 Houxi	*Yangweimai* TE-5 Waiguan	*Renmai* LU-7 Lieque	*Yinweimai* PC-6 Neiguan
Foot	*Yangqiaomai* BL-62 Shenmai	*Daimai* GB-41 Linqi	*Yinqiaomai* KI-6 Zhaohai	*Chongmai* SP-4 Gongsun

The four *Group Luo points* (the French *Group Luo-Passage*) are bilateral, two on the inside and outside of the forearm, and two on the inside and outside leg. Each one harvests the energy of the three main *Yin* or *Yang* upper or lower channels. It is important to test them before other specific points, as finding positivity in just one of them will indicate three of the possible Main Channels implicated in the energetic imbalance and will allow the other nine to be excluded. For example, if point PC-5 Jianshi (group Luo on the *Yin* channels of the upper limb) tests positive, the next step will be to research the therapeutic potential of the points located on three *Yin* channels of the upper limb: *Lung, Pericardium* and *Heart*.

TABLE 3.2 THE 4 GROUP LUO POINTS

3 Hand Yang	*3 Foot Yang*	*3 Hand Yin*	*3 Foot Yin*
TE-8 Sanyangluo	GB-39 Xuanzhong	PC-5 Jianshi	SP-6 Sanyinjiao

The 15 *Luo Connecting points* (*Meridian Luo-Passage* for French authors) are the specific action points on every single channel, as the Luo Collateral Channel starts from these, branching off on one side to the surface thus allowing the excess Qi to be diverted and freed when blocked. On the other side it connects to the channel of the opposite nature.

TABLE 3.3 THE 15 LUO CONNECTING POINTS

Luo Points	Channel	Full	Empty
LU-7 Lieque	Large Intestine	Hot palms and fever	Shortness of breath, frequent urination
HT-5 Tongli	Small Intestine	Fullness in the chest	Language difficulties
PC-6 Neiguan	Triple Energiser	Cardiac pain	Restlessness
SI-7 Zhizheng	Heart	Motor difficulties	Verrucas
LI-6 Pianli	Lung	Odontalgia, deafness	Tooth sensitivity to cold, fullness in chest
TE-5 Waiguan	Pericardium	Spasms in the forearm	Asthenia of the forearm
BL-58 Feiyang	Kidney	Rhinitis, lumbalgia and headache	Epistaxis
GB-37 Guangming	Liver	Syncope	Flaccid paralysis (wei syndrome)
ST-40 Fenglong	Spleen	Sore throat, aphonia, mania	Foot drop
SP-4 Gongsun	Stomach	Abdominal pain, diarrhoea	Oedema
KI-4 Dazhong	Bladder	Restlessness, dysuria	Lumbar pain
LR-5 Ligou	Gall Bladder	Uterine prolapse, hernia	Genital pruritis
CV-15 Jiuwei	Abdomen	Abdominal pain	Pruritis of the abdominal region
GV-1 Changqiang	Head	Vertebral rigidity	Dizziness, heavy head
SP-21 Dabao	Hypochondrium	General pain	General Asthenia

Of special importance is point SP-21 Dabao, which provides access to a fine Qi reticulum enveloping the body like a spider's web: the Great Luo of the Spleen. The Luo points of the individual channels will be tested if the group points show positive results, and if the symptom is located in the area of the channels to which they belong.

The four *Regional Command points* are points which have traditionally been used to therapeutically influence four areas of the body: the face and mouth, the head and neck, the abdomen and the back. They can be tested for symptoms localised in one of these areas.

TABLE 3.4 THE 4 REGIONAL COMMAND POINTS

Abdomen	Back	Face & mouth	Head & neck
ST-36 Zusanli	BL-40 Weizhong	LI-4 Hegu	LU-7 Lieque

The *Tendomuscular Hui points* (Convergence of the Tendomuscular Channels) are indicated for the treatment of dermatosis, neuralgia and muscular problems. They are worth testing since they exercise group control over the three tendomuscular *Yin* or *Yang* channels of the hands and feet, but opinions vary as to how many points should be tested.

TABLE 3.5 THE 3 YANG (YIN) TENDOMUSCULAR MERIDIANS OF THE ARM (LEG)

Yang Arm TM 3	Yin TM 3 Arm	Yang TM 3 Leg	Yin TMM 3 Leg
GB-13 Benshen	GB-22 Yuanye	ST-3 Juliao	CV-2 Qugu
ST-8 Touwei	/	SI-18 Quanliao	CV-3 Zhongji

The five *Shu Transporting points* (French *Shu-Ancient*) are those with the greatest therapeutic value. They are divided into Yuan-Source points and Element points. There are six for each *Yang* channel and five for each *Yin* channel, because the Yuan-Source *Yang* point has only one function, while on the *Yin* channel it also functions as an element point. The Yuan-Source points are considered to be a group on their own and will be discussed shortly. Every element point has the properties of one of the five elements of the doctrine of energy: *fire, earth, metal, water* and *wood*. Points that have general reinforcing or dispersing properties are to be tested when the corresponding channel is believed to be full or empty of Qi. The element organ points (e.g. Lung–Metal) are italicised in the table. The Mother–Son rule should be applied to them in accordance with the generative cycle: [M]other tones, [S]on disperses. The *seasonal* reinforcing and dispersing points (without a table) are to be tested for the same indications, but during one of the five seasons of the Chinese calendar, according to which each is controlled by one of the 5 natural elements: *Spring*–Wood, *Summer*–Fire, *End of Summer*–Earth, *Autumn*–Metal and *Winter*–Water. The fifth season, *End of Summer*, lies between Summer and Autumn. Illnesses sometimes exhibit a seasonal cyclicity and it is not unusual for a patient to come to the surgery for the same or a similar problem, or for one which is completely different, *at the same time of year* as when he first visited. The five Shu Transporting points should also be tested for symptoms of a cyclic nature, like pollen allergies or seasonal ailments (springtime ulcers, winter bronchitis, etc.).

TABLE 3.6 THE 5 SHU TRANSPORTING POINTS

Yin Channel	*Jing–Pozzo (Wood–Spring)*	*Ying–Zampillo (Fire–Summer)*	*Shu–Ruscello (Earth–End of Summer)*	*Jing–River (Metal–Autumn)*	*He–Sea (Water–Winter)*
Lung	LU-11 Shaoshang	LU-10 Yuji	LU-9 Taiyuan – **[M]**	***LU-8 Jingqu***	LU-5 Chize – **[S]**
Pericardium	PC-9 Zhongchong – **[M]**	***PC-8 Laogong***	PC-7 Daling – **[S]**	PC-5 Jianshi	PC-3 Quze
Heart	HT-9 Shaochong – **[M]**	***HT-8 Shaofu***	HT-7 Shenmen – **[S]**	HT-4 Lingdao	HT-3 Shaohai
Spleen	SP-1 Yinbai	SP-2 Dadu – **[M]**	***SP-3 Taibai***	SP-5 Shangqiu – **[S]**	SP-9 Yinlingquan
Liver	***LR-1 Dadun***	LR-2 Xiangjian – **[S]**	LR-3 Taichong	LR-4 Ximen	LR-8 Ququan – **[M]**
Kidney	KI-1 Yongquan – **[S]**	KI-2 Rangu	KI-3 Taixi	KI-7 Fuliu – **[M]**	***KI-10 Yingu***
Yang Channel	*Jing–Pozzo (Metal–Autumn)*	*Ying–Zampillo (Water–Winter)*	*Shu–Ruscello (Wood–Spring)*	*Jing–River (Fire–Summer)*	*He–Sea (Earth–End of Summer)*

Large Intestine	*LI-1* *Shangyang*	LI-2 Erjiang – [S]	LI-3 Sanjiang	LI-5 Yangxi	LI-11 Quchi – [M]
Triple Energiser	TE-1 Guanchong	TE-2 Yemen	TE-3 Yangchi – [M]	*TE-6* *Zhigou*	TE-10 Tianjing – [S]
Small Intestine	SI-1 Shaoze	SI-2 Qiangu	SI-3 Houxi – [M]	*SI-5* *Yanggu*	SI-8 Xiaohai – [S]
Stomach	ST-45 Lidui – [S]	ST-44 Neiting	ST-43 Xiangu	ST-41 Jiexi – [M]	*ST-36* *Zusanli*
Gall Bladder	GB-44 Qiaoyin	GB-43 Xiaxi – [M]	*GB-41* *Linqi*	GB-38 Yangfu – [S]	GB-34 Yanglingquan
Bladder	BL-67 Zhiyin – [M]	*BL-66* *Tonggu*	BL-65 Shugu – [S]	BL-60 Kunlun	BL-40 Weizhong

The 12 *Yuan-Source points* belong to the Shu Transporting points and link the main channel with its corresponding internal organ, passing through the energy of the Upper, Middle and Lower Energiser. Electronic investigation of these points has often highlighted the channel's charge indicator function. Tradition suggests their use in relation to diseases of the organs, especially the *Yin* organs, and they should be tested for all visceral disorders.

TABLE 3.7 THE 12 YUAN-SOURCE POINTS

Lung	LU-9 Taiyuan	Bladder	BL-64 Jinggu
Large Intestine	LI-4 Hegu	Kidney	KI-3 Taixi
Stomach	ST-42 Chongyang	Pericardium	PC-7 Daling
Spleen	SP-3 Taibai	Triple Energiser	TE-4 Yangchi
Heart	HT-7 Shenmen	Gall Bladder	GB-40 Qiuxu
Small Intestine	SI-4 Wangu	Liver	LR-3 Taichong

The 12 *Back Shu or Back Transporting points* (French *Shu-Assent*) are on the dorsal route of the Bladder Channel, and are 'spy' points relating to the energetic wellbeing of the channel-organ or of its function. Their

exploration by means of the Active Points Test is invaluable, as they may reveal information about their respective dermatomes. Indeed, they often correspond to the quick choice *paravertebral points* (see above). The works of numerous authors, particularly Quaglia Senta,[47] pioneer of modern acupuncture in Italy, have led to the recognition of a correlation between Back Shu points and functions of the vegetative nervous system.

TABLE 3.8 THE 12 BACK SHU OR BACK TRANSPORTING POINTS

T3-T4	BL-13	Feishu	Lung
T4-T5	BL-14	Jueyinshu	Pericardium
T5-T6	BL-15	Xinshu	Heart
T6-T7	BL-16	Dushu	*Dumai*
T7-T8	BL-17	Geshu	*Diaphragm*
T8-T9	Extra	Weiwanxiashu	*Epigastrium-Cardia*
T9-T10	BL-18	Ganshu	Liver
T10-T11	BL-19	Danshu	Gall Bladder
T11-T12	BL-20	Pishu	Spleen
T12-L1	BL-21	Weishu	Stomach
L1-L2	BL-22	Sanjiaoshu	Triple Energiser
L2-L3	BL-23	Shenshu	Kidneys
L3-L4	BL-24	Qihaishu	*Peritoneum-Qihai*
L4-L5	BL-25	Dachangshu	Large Intestine
L5-S1	BL-26	Guanyuanshu	*Guanyuan*
foro S1	BL-27	Xiaochangshu	Small Intestine
foro S2	BL-28	Pangguangshu	Bladder
foro S3	BL-29	Zhonglüshu	*Sacrum*
foro S4	BL-30	Baihuanshu	*Prostate-Skene's Glands*

Note that there are 19 points in the complete series of Back Shu points, as shown in Table 3.8 above, but only 12 refer to the main meridians and related organs.

The 12 *Front Mu Collecting points* (*Mu-Herald or Sentinel*) are in some ways similar to the Back Shu points. They are on the front of the chest and belong to the Lung, Stomach, Gall Bladder and Liver Channels, as well as to the *Renmai* Extraordinary Channel. They should be tested in relation to visceral diseases and locoregional symptoms caused by these diseases, such as cough, gastric pain and colic, hiccups, vomiting, etc.

TABLE 3.9 THE 12 FRONT MU COLLECTING POINTS

Lung	LU-1 Zhongfu	Bladder	CV-3 Zhongji
Large Intestine	ST-25 Tianshu	Kidney	GB-25 Jingmen
Stomach	CV-12 Zhongwan	Pericardium	CV-17 Shanzhong
Spleen	LR-13 Zhangmen	Triple Energiser	CV-5 Shimen
Heart	CV-14 Jujue	Gall Bladder	GB-25 Riyue
Small Intestine	CV-4 Guanyuan	Liver	LR-14 Qimen

The 16 *Xi Cleft*[j] or *Accumulation points* (French *Xi–Urgency* and Japanese *geki*): there is a given Xi point for every Main and Extraordinary Channel, with the exception of the *Dumai* and *Renmai* Channels. According to tradition, these points are located at a greater depth than the others. Here *blood* and *energy* converge. They can even improve energy and blood circulation in the channel itself, as well as being traditionally indicated, and therefore suitable for testing, in acute diseases that affect the Main Channel and its related organ.

TABLE 3.10 THE 16 XI CLEFT OR ACCUMULATION POINTS

Lung	LU-6 Kongzui	Bladder	BL-63 Jinmen
Large Intestine	LI-7 Wenliu	Kidney	KI-5 Shuiquan
Stomach	ST-34 Liangqiu	Pericardium	PC-4 Ximen
Spleen	SP-8 Diji	Triple Heater	TE-7 Huizong
Heart	HT-6 Yinxi	Gall Bladder	GB-36 Waiqiu
Small Intestine	SI-6 Yanglao	Liver	LR-6 Zhongdu
Yangqiaomai	BL-59 Fuyang	Yinqiaomai	KI-8 Jiaoxin
Yangweimai	GB-35 Yangjiao	Yinweimai	KI-9 Zhubin

---

j　　Deep crack, slit, chasm

The eight *Hui Influential* or *Gathering points* (*Hui-Meeting*) are situated on the course of more than one channel and have a general effect on various organs and functions. They are very useful for the Test, in particular the first three in the list.

TABLE 3.11 THE 8 HUI INFLUENTIAL OR GATHERING POINTS

LR-13 Zhangmen	*Zang* viscera
CV-12 Zhongwan	*Fu* organs
CV-17 Shanzhong	Qi – breath
BL-17 Geshu	Blood
GB-34 Yanglingquan	Tendons
BL-11 Dazhu	Bones
GB-39 Xuanzhong	Marrow
LU-9 Taiyuan	Pulses (arteries)

The ten *Window of Sky points* (page 96): even though no source material in English mentions this group, Deadman and Al-Khafaji acknowledge the indications that would explain it:[48] all *Jue* Qi disorders (the so-called rebel Qi), with alterations or blockages in the flow of blood or energy between the thorax and the head. These points should definitely be tested in relation to sudden symptoms affecting the neck and head (we have seen the use of ST-9 Renyin for acute lumbalgia), all sensory disorders (deafness, anosmia etc.), vomiting and diarrhoea. The following list is taken from a single source and is not exhaustive.[49]

TABLE 3.12 THE 10 WINDOW OF SKY POINTS

LU-3 Tianfu	Asthma, epistaxis, brachialgia
LI-18 Futu	Cough, catarrh, sore throat
ST-9 Renyin	Hypertension, asthma, pharyngitis, aphasia
SI-16 Tianchuang	Deafness, tinnitus, sore throat, stiffness and contracture of the neck
SI-17 Tianrong	Tonsillitis, sore throat, aphasia
SI-18 Quanliao	Facial paralysis, odontalgia, trigeminal neuralgia
BL-10 Tianzhu	Occipital headache, locked and stiff neck, insomnia, pharyngitis
PC-1 Tianchi	Chest oppression, pain in the hypochondrium, adenopathies
TE-16 Tianyou	Deafness, stiff neck
GV-16 Fengfu	Cold, headache, mental diseases, apoplexy

The 12 *Entry–Exit points* of the Ordinary and Extraordinary Channels do not have the same value as the Luo or Source points. Through them, the Extraordinary Channels connect with the Main Channels. They are to be tested if the opening points show indifferent results.

TABLE 3.13 THE 12 ENTRY–EXIT POINTS

Entry	LU-1	LI-4	ST-1	SP-1	HT-1	SI-1	BL-1	KI-1	PC-1	TE-1	GB-1	LR-1
Exit	LU-7	LI-20	ST-42	SP-21	HT-9	SI-19	BL-67	KI-22	PC-8	TE-22	GB-41	LR-14

The 12 *Chinese Hours points* (French *Pen–time* points[k]), among the five *Transporting Shu* points, are those which have the same characteristics as the natural element of the channel to which they belong. So LU-8 Jingqu is the metal point of the Lung Channel, an organ which is the equivalent to the element metal, LR-1 Dadun is the wood point of the Liver Channel, an organ which is the equivalent to the element wood, etc. These points are called 'time' points because their activity is more intense when the channel is in the hour of maximum energy according to Chinese time. According to traditional Chinese doctrine, the Qi

---

k   These points could be considered a French exclusive. I have not been able to find anything about them in English either on paper or on the internet.

completes one circuit lap of the main channels in 24 hours, and stops flowing in each channel for 1 of the 12 hours in the Chinese day (one Chinese hour is the equivalent to two of ours). Each organ is considered to be at maximum energy level during its own particular hour and is therefore in the best possible condition for stimulating. Twelve hours later the same channel is considered to be at the minimum energy level and in the best possible condition for dispersal or sedation. The time points can be tested when the symptom manifests during the particular hour belonging to the channel concerned.

TABLE 3.14 THE 12 CHINESE HOURS POINTS

Yin Hour	03–05	Lung	LU-8 Jingqu	metal points
Mao Hour	05–07	Large Intestine	LI-1 Shangyang	
Zhen Hour	07–09	Stomach	ST-36 Zusanli	earth points
Su Hour	09–11	Spleen	SP-3 Taibai	
Wu Hour	11–13	Heart	HT-8 Shaofu	fire points
Wei Hour	13–15	Small Intestine	SI-5 Yanggu	
Shen Hour	15–17	Bladder	BL-66 Tonggu	water points
Yu Hour	17–19	Kidney	KI-10 Yingu	
Xu Hour	19–21	Pericardium	PC-8 Laogong	fire points
Hai Hour	21–23	Triple Heater	TE-6 Zhigou	
Ci Hour	23–01	Gall Bladder	GB-41 Linqi	wood points
Chu Hour	01–03	Liver	LR-1 Dadun	

The *extra points* are located on the Main and Extraordinary Channels or outside, on their own or in groups. Extra points may be subjected to the Test as well (see Figure 2.22, page 64; Figure 3.12, page 99 and Figure 5.1, page 133). I will never be able to say 'thank you' enough to Royston Low for his book about the extra points in acupuncture,[14] as it has made me realise that the search for therapeutic points does not stop at the canons of tradition (see Figure 3.14, page 101). 387 points are illustrated together with their anatomical location, Chinese names and indications, not counting those of the hand, foot, nose, face and scalp, which on their own belong to the reflex therapy method of treatment. The Ahshi points may also number indirectly among the extra points. Their name originates from the expression of pain 'Ah!'

that the patient gives when the point (shi) is subjected to palpitation. The *Neijing* describes them like this: 'A painful point is an acupuncture point.'[31] The Ahshi points may coincide with local points from the Test's quick choice criterion.

3.5 A FEW MORE WORDS ABOUT PALPATION

Skin palpation is integral to the teaching of both western clinical medicine and traditional acupuncture. It goes without saying that it must be done properly if the Active Points Test is to give valid results. Both local and paravertebral points, as well as the spondyloid points, are explored with both hands using the *pincé roulé* method in accordance with the quick choice criterion, while practitioners of TCM carry out palpation on the Channels in accordance with the reasoned choice criterion. This shows how common it is to find points which are extra painful and therefore active in terms of the Test. Figure 3.11 illustrates longitudinal skin palpation in a centrifugal direction on the Qi current, as part of a search for painful points to test on the Gall Bladder Channel. This relates to a case described later in this book (see Figure 5.8, page 145). Figure 3.13 on the other hand, illustrates transverse palpation in the area of the calf muscle (sural biceps) searching for point BL-57 Chengshan, used in the treatment of haemorrhoids (see Figure 3.10, page 85). The infiltration of cellulite into the tissues and the presence of marks, dilated venules and capillaries, lenticular angiomas, nevi and flat or peduncular verrucas are always significant pointers to energetic disturbances in the channels (blood stagnation, damp, dryness, heat, etc.).

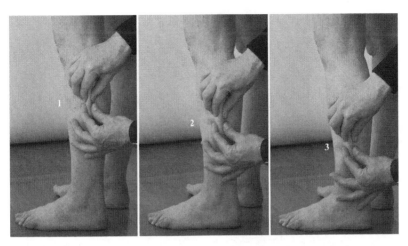

Figure 3.11 Skin palpation of the Gall Bladder Meridian on the leg

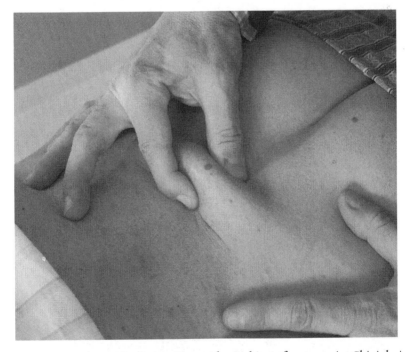

Figure 3.12 The Active Points Test with pinching of extra point Shiqizhui, the seventeenth vertebra, for positional lumbalgia in a prone position
The Chinese counted the vertebrae starting from the first thoracic. Located between the spinal apophyses L5 and S1, it has been marked with a felt-tip pen.

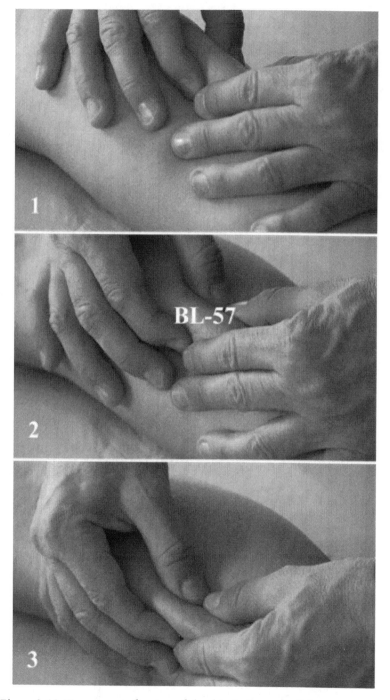

Figure 3.13 Transverse palpation of the skin in the area of the sura

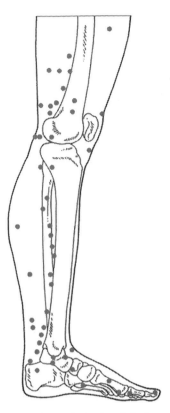

Figure 3.14 Extra points on the medial side of the lower limbs, and on the sole of the foot
(See Low, note 14.)

3.6 AURICULAR PUNCTURE

Auricular puncture is based on the application of different shaped needles, metal pins and vaccaria seeds to the skin of the auricle. It is used as a therapy in its own right or as a complement to acupuncture. Auricular puncture theory postulates that there is a somatotopic relationship between the auricle and an upside-down human foetus (Figure 3.15),[1] with the earlobe corresponding to the cranium, the antihelix to the vertebral column, the cavum conchae to the splanchnic

---

1   'Somatotopic /so·ma·to·top·ic/ (-top´ik) means related to particular areas of the body; describing organisation of motor area of the brain, control of the movement of different parts of the body being centered in specific regions of the cortex.' (Dorland's Medical Dictionary for Health Consumers).

organs and so on, so that any physical activity on the ear points will result in the nervous system provoking a reflex action which will have an effect on the locoregional or general symptom. Thus the shoulder and cervical rachis points will be used for scapulo-humeral periarthritis, the liver and allergy points for pruritus, etc.

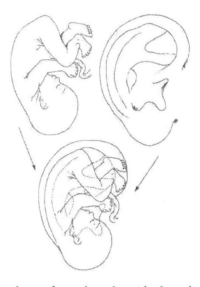

Figure 3.15 Similar shape of auricle and upside-down human foetus

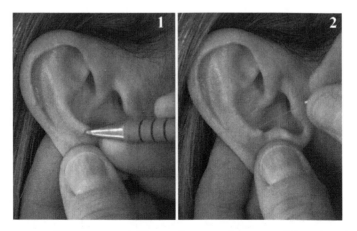

Figure 3.16 The Active Points Test on the auricular point of the cervical area, in relation to a case of cervicobrachialgia on the right side
Execution of test (1) with ballpoint pen, (2) with needle.

The practice established by Paul Nogier,[50] who discovered the methodology, is to explore one ear at a time, beginning with the dominant side, using a spring loaded probe with rounded tip or an electronic detector in the search for painful and particularly sensitive areas. Once the most sensitive areas have been located, needles can be inserted and the appropriate manipulation carried out.

In auricular puncture the Active Points Test is performed before needles are inserted, so as to take advantage of its strong predictive capacity. The nib of an empty biro may be used or the area to be explored may be touched with the tip of a needle (Figure 3.16). It is not necessary to wait for the appearance of a depression mark on the skin as there is very little subcutaneous tissue in the ear, just as there is in the fingertips. The search for reflex zones in the ear may also be carried out using an electronic detector, as it has been demonstrated that cutaneous points show specific resistance changes to the passage of electrical current.

The Test gives excellent results on auricular points as, in the body's defence system against pain and organ dysfunction, the ear is located at a 'higher' level than the rest of the soma, and is nearer to the sensory cortex. For this reason, the control and inhibition of nociceptive afferents (symptoms) coming from spinal and cephalic areas is more effective than for the other areas of the body. In terms of controlling nociception, if we compare the spinal cord (with the somatic points) to the peripheral defences of a castle, such as the moat and the walls, then the thalamus (with the auricular points) corresponds to the citadel and the king's guard, the last and fiercest line of defence (Figure 3.17). At the beginning of an assault (acute disease), if both defensive systems are made to act immediately, the probabilities of fighting off the attack and preventing a siege (chronic disease) will increase. This is a valid reason for linking auricular puncture to classical acupuncture.

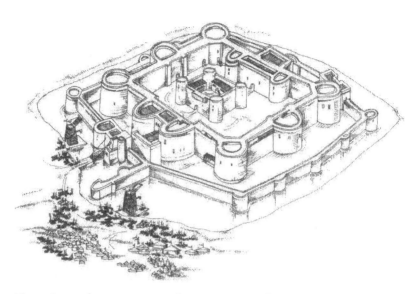

Figure 3.17 The concentric castle suggests an analogy with the different levels in the neuroreflex regulation of nociception

I have found positive points (+, ++) in 113 of the 119 cases in which I have performed the Active Points Test on the ear, that is to say 94.95%. As I am not an auricular puncture 'specialist', in 1995 I sought the detailed opinion of Marco Romoli. A man with an open mind and much clinical experience, he accepted my invitation, making an invaluable contribution and providing a study of 18 patients which is appended to this volume (The Active Points Test in Auricular Punture). With his permission, I will quote the paragraph about the Test from the chapter on auricle examination methods from his *Agopuntura Auricolare* (2003):[36]

> The Needle Contact Test (NCT) was originally proposed in 1995 by the physician Stefano Marcelli who named it the 'Active Point Test'. His intention was to introduce a diagnostic method which could quickly and accurately identify the most effective points for therapy.
>
> The test was used by the author in the case of painful syndromes and required the collaboration of the patient who was asked to keep his attention fully focused on his perception of pain throughout the test. Among the Meridian acupuncture points suitable in the treatment of a given painful condition the

author was able, through his test, to identify the point/s which most reduced the intensity of symptoms. The test was proposed to doctors and physiotherapists and several kinds of stimulation were recommended by the author, among them also acupressure. When a needle was applied to the acupuncture point for a few seconds, it was to touch the skin without penetration. The sensation to be felt by the patient was that of a superficial puncture of such light intensity that it should not cause any bother at all. The best diameter for the testing needle was between 0.25 and 0.35 mm. Especially in case of more widespread pain syndromes, different points were tested following the concepts of harmonization and redistribution of energy in the Meridians which are typical [of] TCM.

Once the Meridian point effective in reducing pain has been identified, the same needle can be inserted into the skin for starting treatment. According to Marcelli the result of the test could be rated as indifferent, negative, moderately and strongly positive. An indifferent answer corresponded to no variation, negative to a worsening of pain and positive when the reduction of pain was more or less rapid and widespread.

Applications of the Needle Contact Test
NCT may be helpful in different conditions. Each of them has a diagnostic phase afterwards completed by therapeutic intervention.

The main applications are for pain conditions of whatever origin and for symptoms related to the locomotor system such as myofascial pain and stiffness with reduced range of motion.

The different applications examined to date are:

1. for current pain

2. for migraine attack

3. for pain on palpation of tender points/areas

4. for pain provoked by movement

5. for deactivating Myofascial Trigger Points and improving the range of motion

6. for muscular hypertonus: our experiences in the craniomandibular disorders.

3.7 MESOTHERAPY

Mesotherapy is a technique of injecting medical cocktails, usually procaine or lidocaine and other allopathic or homeopathic drugs diluted with a saline solution in the ratio of 1:10. Special instruments are used: short needles (0.30–0.40 mm x 4-6-13), multi-injectors and automatic pistols (Figure 3.18). The advantages of this therapy are that it combines the actions of puncture, bleeding, anaesthetic and other drugs, which reinforce each other and often give immediate and lasting results. Devised by Dr Michel Pistor in the 1950s, its practice has become more and more widespread in Europe and throughout the world. Mesotherapy consists essentially of *localised microinjections* and *nappage*. The former are administered intradermally or subcutaneously, in painful points or in points which are located on the orthogonal projection of the problem that requires treatment. The latter consists of tapping larger areas with a short needle, pressing simultaneously on the piston of the syringe to deliver the drugs.

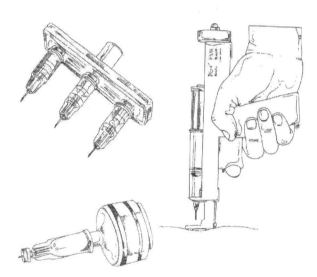

Figure 3.18 Mesotherapy instruments: three-needle linear multi-injector, shortened needle for nappage and Den' Hub mechanical pistol

Mesotherapy is an elective therapy for pathologies occurring locoregionally, whose indications range from the field of rheumatology to that of aesthetic medicine, particularly in the treatment of cellulite.

Most mesotherapists administer microinjections not only in local points, but also in those which are further away from the seat of the pathology but related to it according to the concepts of reflexology[51, 52] and traditional Chinese acupuncture.

Mesopuncture, injections of allopathic drugs into acupuncture points, was advanced as a therapy at the beginning of the 1980s, but with very little following. The injection of homogeneous homeopathic remedies into acupuncture points suggested by Ballesteros,[23] is still supported today by Le Coz for the treatment of muscle pathology.[53] The injection of complex homeopathic remedies can only weaken the rationale of a methodology which already has more than one reliable mode of action. This is a personal opinion, and in medicine Paracelsus's aphorism is always true: 'He who cures is right!'

Mesotherapists can make use of the Active Points Test, referring to the quick choice criterion on *local, paravertebral* and *spondyloid* points for direction. Those mesotherapists who are familiar with acupuncture points will be able to test the points they choose according to the reasoned choice criterion.

In this paragraph from the first edition of this book I suggested that mesotherapists should test points with an acupuncture needle, adding:

> I want to emphasise…that it is not at all rare to observe a symptom, which is only alleviated when an acupuncture point is tested with a needle, disappear completely while pinching the area where the point is located, since the surface area affected by the neurosensory stimulation of the 'pinch' is much larger than that of the point itself and may therefore prove to be more active as a whole.

I was setting out in a nutshell the simplest version of the Test to date. Further suggestions on what action to take will be given later, in the section which deals with post-Test therapy. In conclusion, let us consider the opinion of Multedo, one of the most well-known French mesotherapists and my own teacher:

> For my part, I have begun to use it successfully in relation to certain common conditions, such as sciatic or cervicobrachial neuralgia. It allows us to know if we should treat or not treat, if we should inject without hesitation or not inject a product that could be

uselessly painful; hence the advantages are that it is effective and saves time. I therefore believe that Dr Marcelli's method should be incorporated into our therapeutic practices *in so far as we consider mesotherapy to constitute not just a simple form of local therapy but also a form of 'wet reflex therapy'*.

3.8 NEURAL THERAPY

Neural therapy is a technique of German origin devised in 1925 by the brothers Ferdinand and Walter Huneke and practised a great deal in English-speaking countries.[29] It is based on the injection of the local anaesthetic *procaine*, with or without caffeine, in the dermis or near the peripheral nerves and into ganglions. Its aim is the neutralisation of afference caused by the disorder, and its main indications are diseases of the musculoskeletal and neurovegetative systems. It includes intradermal and subcutaneous injections (papules), which go by the name of *segmental therapy*,[m] and deep injections which penetrate as far as the peritoneum or the suprarenal pole with the purpose of treating deep ganglions. It is also used for the neutralisation of so-called *interference fields*, the inflammatory 'chronic foci' (pulpitis and dental granuloma, tonsillitis, appendicitis, salpingitis etc.) and the cicatricial 'foci' which are of either traumatic or surgical origin, considered responsible for the genesis and retention of various disorders. If a cause and effect relationship really exists between the suspicious 'focus' and the distal pathology, such as chronic articular pain for example, the injection of procaine produces *Sekundenphänomen*,[n] that is to say the disappearance of the symptom in a second. Another way of administering therapy is the rapid intravenous bolus, used primarily for the treatment of headaches.

Neural therapy can make use of the Active Points Test in accordance with the rapid choice criterion. *Local, paravertebral* and *spondyloid* points may in this way become the favoured first site for injections of procaine. As will be seen from the section dealing with therapy, neural therapy is considered to be a remarkably effective medium for soothing the very few points which respond negatively to the Test.

---

m   Here *segment* is a synonym of dermatome.

n   The second phenomenon.

3.9 WESTERN MANUAL THERAPIES

Methodologies belonging to this group are manual treatments of western origin, ranging from physiotherapeutic massotherapy to Dicke's connective tissue massage, Rolfing and myofascial release therapy, from Maigne's vertebral manipulation to osteopathy and chiropractice. Here too the Active Points Test can be used to point to a diagnosis. As these methodologies have little to do with TCM, the rapid choice criterion is useful both for pain and for functional limitations to the locomotive apparatus, where it can help to decide which vertebral level to work on.

3.10 MEDICAL HISTORY AND BLIND ACUPUNCTURE

Western medicine first of all, and then TCM, have taught me that, from conception to disintegration, our bodies complete the journey with their baggage full of predispositions: to health as regards some organs and to disease as regards others. Observing myself and patients over the course of the years, I have ascertained that these predispositions do not change easily, and that organs and systems preserve the same relationship of strength and weakness, even though it may lessen with age and the occurrence of major events. The means common to both forms of medicine for investigating these predispositions is an interview with the patient to discuss any illnesses he or she may have suffered. In western medicine this is known as the *medical history* of past illness.

I have already explained how, beginning with the therapeutic activity of point ST-38 Tiaokou, making the link between past and present stomach problems in patients who benefited from puncture of that point was fundamental for devising the Test. For this reason I suggest considering the possibility that symptoms which the patient is suffering from today may constitute a different form of expression of a past illness that was apparently cured. The remarkable power of modern drugs to counteract all sorts of disorders must be taken into account, and the symptoms 'subtracted' by drugs from the overall disease reduction should be added to the ongoing symptomatology. A patient who is taking proton pump inhibitors no longer suffers from a burning sensation in the stomach, but that suppressed 'heat' could have moved to the shoulder. A patient taking diuretics has an 'assisted spleen' but the damp suppressed, for example, by the lungs (through cardiac insufficiency) might have moved into the knees. Any homeopaths reading this would accuse me of stating the obvious.

The fact that the same organs and systems have a tendency to suffer from illness over time is also linked with spontaneous and surgical trauma. During the examination of patients' skin before inserting the needles, I have often found – and now it is the neural therapists'[29] turn to be happy – traumatic and surgical scars next to or in the vicinity of points and on channels that I was on the verge of choosing. Despite being very wary of the superstitious aspects of TCM and the blind faith of some followers and teachers, I came up with the idea that the *latent awareness of the active point* might be extended to the channels. The *latent awareness of the active channel* would make the 'suffering' channel, and no other, predisposed to natural trauma. A channel might be overly full of blood, and so the patient might injure a finger, apparently 'by accident'. I have happened to cut my index finger (Large Intestine meridian) 'inadvertently' many times after eating too much meat, and have seen the same thing happen to others. I have seen scars from cuts to the middle finger (Triple Energiser meridian) in women with dysmenorrhea or suffering from a difficult menopause, wounds to the forehead and nose (lung-linked areas) in children suffering from chronic heat diseases of the throat and the bronchial tube, and much more besides. From a scientific point of view, this is not the proper time and place for a fascinating discussion of hypotheses that are better suited to a conversation at a dinner party, but it might be worth looking again at traumatology in the light of the theory of Qi and the Channels. The type of pain in the Channels creates a predisposition to various types of trauma: so, if an excess of blood predisposes towards or even 'tries to find' a bleeding wound, a Qi deficiency in a particular Channel could 'invoke' a contusion or a fracture, and an invasion of cold could cause a burn. I have called this phenomenon 'blind acupuncture'. The aim of these considerations is to persuade the reader to put to the Test points chosen on Channels that have already been affected in the past by trauma, for which scars are visible.

I would like to reflect briefly on the medical history of illnesses which have thankfully been treated through surgery. The surgical removal of gall stones puts an end to colics, but does not solve the cause of the problem (cold, dryness, catarrh etc.) which thickens bile and encourages salt precipitation. Unless there are critical changes in diet and behaviour, years later the patient's bile will have thickened again, and the surgical history will give an indication as to a reasonable series of points that should be tested. This may be taken to apply to the majority of surgical pathologies, with due consideration for the differences between individual cases.

3.11 DURATION OF THE TEST (HOW MANY POINTS SHOULD BE FOUND ACTIVE)

During the first evening presentation of the Active Points Test to colleagues of the Associazione Medici Agopuntori Bolognesi (or Fondazione Matteo Ricci), Dr Giovanardi asked how many the active points, both positive and negative, needed to be found in order for an appropriate therapy to be carried out. I gave an answer which is still true today.

A traditional acupuncturist, a chiropractor and a mesotherapist will all behave differently. While the first may use the Test to confirm whether the points chosen according to the eight rules, and pulse and tongue examination are really 'active', for the others the Test may be a tool of prime importance for the diagnosis. If the Test has shown that a single point is enough to eliminate the patient's symptom, that point will be enough for the therapy. On the other hand, if it has indicated more points with weaker positivity which are each incapable of eliminating the disorder when punctured individually, it is likely that simultaneous puncture will strengthen the effect. Successive sessions will indicate whether other points should be tested or 'treated' or whether the medical protocol should remain unaltered.

In general, the search for the active points will stop at five or six units. This will be enough, particularly if they are not only local points but also belong to groups which are traditionally endowed with great therapeutic value, such as the *Transporting Shu* points.

3.12 ACUPOINT FORMULAS

There now follows an overview of the principle affections for which the Active Points Test is indicated, with the relevant acupoint *formulas*. I cannot repeat often enough that the Test must be executed at a time when the patient's symptom is present, and care should be taken to look for possible movements and positions that aggravate it. I personally take advantage of every opportunity when a symptom is ongoing to use the rapid choice criterion. It is always interesting for us as practitioners and for the patients to discover that we possess a simple instrument for guiding therapy: *sensitivity*.

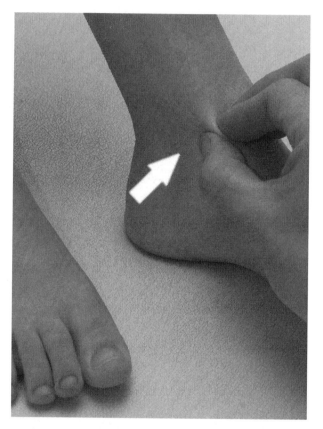

Figure 3.19 The Active Points Test on point LR-4 Zhongfeng for dysphonia
This symptom is not traditionally among the specific indications for this point. The patient was invited to talk while the point was being pinched and then touched by the needle, and to report any changes in the symptom.

For every symptom listed I have suggested a few of the *Local points* traditionally considered to be the most effective, and the main and Extraordinary Channels where the distal points for the Test should be searched for using the *palper rouler* method. It is precisely at the distal points that the illness shows its character, determining often original combinations of the 'active points' (Figure 3.19). Let us be clear: there is no such thing as a 'formula' which is effective every time. It should be remembered that points in the head area cannot be considered local points, and *if points on the feet treat the head, then points on the head treat the feet.*

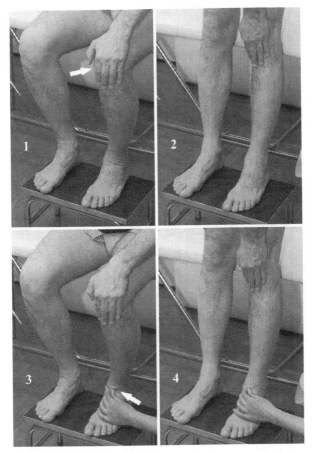

Figure 3.20 Execution of the Test for 'cracking' in the knee joint, already treated with injections of hyaluronic acid

The most painful point during palpation, which later proved to the most effective in eliminating the symptom, was ST-41 Jiexi, a fire point on the Stomach Channel. The hypomobility of the knee numbers among this point's secondary indications. (1) Resting the hand on the bent knee so as to feel the cracking. (2) Extending the leg. (3) Identifying the most painful point. (4) Eliminating the symptom. It is worth noting that the patient was suffering from gastritis, which is a main indication of point ST-41.

The search for the *distal* active points (Figure 3.20) is necessary when dealing with channels that are considered to be the cause of a given symptom, like the lung and kidney channels in cases of dyspnoea. Nevertheless, the indication does not exclude the possibility of finding positive points on other previously unsuspected energy paths.

Respiratory system, pharynx and throat
RHINITIS AND SINUSITIS

> *Local points:* EX-1 Yintang (see Figure 2.22, page 64), EX-3 Yuyao, EX Bitong, EX Neiyingxiang, EX Shangyingxiang, BL-1 Jingming, BL-2 Zanzhu, LI-20 Yingxiang
>
> *Channels: Dumai, Chongmai,* Lung and Large Intestine, Liver, Kidney, Pericardium

ASTHMA, COUGH

> *Local points:* CV-17 Shanzhong, LU-1 Zhongfu, LU-2 Yunmen, KI-26 Yuzhong, KI-27 Shufu
>
> *Channels: Renmai, Chongmai,* Lung, Large Intestine, Liver, Bladder and Gall Bladder

DYSPHONIA AND APHONIA

> *Local points:* ST-9 Renyin, ST-10 Shuitu, LI-17 Tianding. All 'Window of the Sky' points
>
> *Channels: Renmai, Chongmai,* Lung, Large Intestine, Stomach, Spleen, Liver (see Figure 3.19, page 112)

PHARYNGEAL AND TRACHEAL PAIN, TONSILLITIS

> *Local points:* ST-9 Renyin, ST-10 Shuitu, CV-17 Shanzhong, LU-1 Zhongfu, LU-2 Yunmen, EX-11 Zengyin, CV-20 Huagai, CV-21 Xuanji, CV-22 Tiantu
>
> *Channels: Renmai, Yinweimai, Chongmai,* Lung, Large Intestine, Kidney

Chewing and digestive system
TOOTHACHE – TOP ARCH

> *Local points:* ST-2 Sibai, ST-3 Juliao, ST-7 Xiaguan, SI-18 Quanliao, SI-19 Tinggong, TE-21 Ermen, GB-2 Tinghui, LI-19

Heliao, LI-20 Yingxiang, EX Neiyingxiang, EX Shangyingxiang, GV-26 Renzhong, GV-27 Duiduan, GV-28 Yinjiao

Channels: *Dumai, Chongmai, Yangweimai*, Large Intestine, Stomach, Bladder

TOOTHACHE – BOTTOM ARCH

Local points: ST-4 Dicang, ST-5 Daying, ST-6 Jiache, CV-24 Chengjiang, CV-24 Bis, EX-5 Jiachengjiang

Channels: *Renmai, Chongmai, Yinweimai*, Stomach, Large Intestine

GASTRODUODENAL PAIN AND ULCER

Local points: CV-9 Shuifen, CV-12 Zhongwan, CV-13 Shangwan, CV-15 Jiuwei, KI-19 Yindu, KI-20 Tonggu, KI-20 Chengman, ST-21 Liangmen

Channels: *Renmai, Chongmai*, Stomach, Large Intestine, Heart, Gall Bladder

APPENDICULAR PAIN AND COLITIS

Local points: ST-25 Tiantu, ST-26 Wailing, ST-30 Qichong, ST-15 Daheng, KI-15 Zhongzhu, KI-16 Huangshu, CV-4 Guanyuan, CV-5 Shimen, CV-6 Qihai

Channels: *Chongmai, Daimai, Renmai*, Large Intestine, Stomach, Small Intestine, Gall Bladder, Liver

HAEMORRHOIDS (PRURITUS, FEELING OF HEAVINESS AND PAIN CAUSED BY CONTRACTING THE ANAL SPHINCTER)

Local points: GV-1 Changqiang, BL-35 Huiyang, CV-6 Qihai

Channels: *Dumai, Chongmai, Renmai*, Large Intestine, Stomach, Liver

Genito-urinary system
KIDNEY AND URETHRAL PAIN

Local points: BL-23 Shenshu, KI-16 Huangshu, LR-13 Zhangmen, GB-25 Jingmen

Channels: *Chongmai, Daimai, Yinweimai*, Kidney, Bladder

BLADDER PAIN AND CYSTITIS

Local points: CV-2 Qugu, CV-3 Zhongji, CV-4 Guanyuan, CV-6 Qihai, KI-11 Henggu, CV-12 Dahe, ST-29 Guilai, ST-30 Chongmai

Channels: Chongmai, Renmai, Daimai, Bladder, Kidney, Spleen

PELVIC PAIN AND ADNEXITIS

Local points: CV-2 Qugu, CV-3 Zhongji, CV-4 Guanyuan, CV-6 Qihai, KI-11 Henggu, CV-12 Dahe, ST-29 Guilai, ST-30 *Chongmai,* LR-10 Wuli, LR-11 Yinlian, LR-12 Jimai

Channels: Chongmai, Renmai, Kidney, Liver, Pericardium

Cardiocirculatory system

ALTERATIONS IN CARDIAC RHYTHMN, CHEST PAIN, PALPITATION AND ANGINA PECTORIS

Local points: CV-17 Shanzhong, KI-22 Bulang, KI-23 Shenfeng, KI-24 Lingxu, HE-1 Jiquan, PC-1 Tianchi, SP-21 Dabao, ST-18 Rugen, ST-19 Burong

Channels: Renmai, Yinweimai, Chongmai, Heart, Small Intestine, Stomach, Pericardium, Spleen

SUPERFICIAL PHLEBITIS AND THROMBOPHLEBITIS

Local points: Search for the active points through careful pinching of painful areas, also through the use of a pointscope, near to the adventitia of the vessel concerned as well as: SP-6 Sanyinjiao, SP-9 Yinlingquan, BL-40 Weizhong, LR-7 Xiguan, LR-8 Ququan, ST-30 *Chongmai,* LR-10 Wuli, LR-11 Yinlian, LR-12 Jimai

Channels: Chongmai, Yinqiaomai, Yinweimai, Kidney, Liver, Spleen, Bladder

HYPOTENSION, CIRCULATORY ASTHENIA

Local points: LU-9 Taiyuan, KI-3 Taixi, PC-6 Neiguan

Channels: Chongmai, Dumai, Yangweimai, Stomach, Pericardium

Locomotive system

Ample space is dedicated to the locomotive system because of the excellent results achieved with it using the Active Points Test.

MYALGIA

Local points: With a pointscope, search for points near the painful muscular region as well as points located on the proximal and distal insertions.

Channels: Tendino Muscular Meridians (TMM), Stomach, Bladder

ACUTE AND CHRONIC STIFF NECK

Local points: GV-14 Dazhui, GV-15 Yamen, GV-16 Fengfu, BL-10 Tianzhu, BL-11 Dazhu, GB-20 Fengchi, CV-24 Chengjiang, EX-17 Dingchuan, EX-18 Wuming, EX-26 Luozhen, EX Hinshi, EX Bailao

Channels: Dumai, Renmai, Large Intestine, Small Intestine, Bladder, Triple Heater, *Yangqiaomai*

CERVICAL AND CERVICOBRACHIAL PAIN

Local points: GV-14 Dazhui, GV-15 Yamen, GV-16 Fengfu, BL-10 Tianzhu, BL-11 Dazhu, GB-20 Fengchi, GB-21 Jianjing, TE-15 Tianliao, SI-14 Jianwaishu, SI-15 Jianzhongshu, EX-17 Dingchuan, EX-18 Wuming, EX Xinshi, EX Bailao

Channels: Dumai, Yangqiaomai, Bladder, Large Intestine, Small Intestine, Triple Heater, Gall Bladder

SHOULDER PAIN

Local points: The same points as those used for cervical pain as well as LU-1 Zhongfu, LU-2 Yumen, EX Xiaokuai, EX-22 Jianzhong, LI-13 Wuli, LI-14 Binao, LI-15 Jianyu, LI-16 Jugu, SI-9 Jianzhen, SI-10 Naoshu, SI-11 Tianzong, TE-13 Naohui, TE-14 Jianliao

Channels: Yangqiaomai, Yangweimai, Stomach (ST-38 Tiaokou), Small Intestine, Large Intestine, Triple Heater, Gall Bladder

TENNIS ELBOW AND GOLFER'S ELBOW

Local points: LI-7 Wenliu, LI-8 Xialian, LI-9 Shanglian, LI-10 Shousanli, LI-11 Quchi, LI-12 Zhouliao, LI-13 Wuli, LU-5 Chize,

SI-6 Yanglao, SI-7 Zhizheng, SI-8 Xiaohai, TE-10 Tianjing, TE-11 Qinglengyuan, HE-3 Shaohai, PC-3 Quze

Channels: Yangweimai, Yinweimai, Large Intestine, Small Intestine, Triple Heater, Gall Bladder

DORSALGIA

Local points: The Shu Transporting Bladder points as well as GV-3 Yaoyangguan, GV-4 Mingmen, GV-5 Xuanshu, GV-6 Jizhong, GV-7 Zhongshu, GV-8 Jinsuo, GV-9 Zhiyang, GV-10 Lingtai, GV-11 Shendao, GV-12 Shenzhu, GV-13 Taodao, EX-18 Wuming, EX-21 Huatuojiaji

Channels: Dumai, Yangqiaomai, Yinqiaomai, Bladder, Kidney, Stomach, Triple Heater

LUMBOSCIATALGIA, DISCAL HERNIA PAIN, SACRALGIA

Local points: The lumbar and sacral Shu Transporting Bladder points as well as GV-3 Yaoyangguan, GV-4 Mingmen, GV-5 Xuanshu, GV-6 Jizhong, EX-21 Huatuojiaji, EX-20 Yaoqi, BL-31 Shangliao, BL-32 Ciliao, BL-33 Zhongliao, BL-34 Xialiao, BL-35 Huiyang, BL-36 V Chengfu

Channels: Dumai, Yangqiaomai, Yinqiaomai, Bladder, Kidney, Stomach, Triple Heater

COCCYGODYNIA

Local points: EX-21 Huatuojiaji, EX-20 Yaoqi, BL-31 Shangliao, BL-32 Ciliao, BL-33 Zhongliao, BL-34 Xialiao, BL-35 Huiyang, BL-36 Chengfu

Channel: Dumai, Yangqiaomai, Yinqiaomai, Bladder, Kidney, Stomach, Triple Heater

COXALGIA

Local points: The same points as for lumbalgia as well as GB-27 Wushu, GV-28 Weidao, GB-29 Juliao, GB-30 Huantiao, GB-31 Fengshi, ST-30 Chongmai, LR-10 Wuli, LR-11 Yinlian, LR-12 Jimai, SP-11 Jimen, SP-12 Chongmen

Channels: Dumai, Yangqiaomai, Gall Bladder, Bladder, Stomach, Kidney

GONALGIA

Local points: ST-32 Futu, ST-33 Yinshi, ST-34 Liangqiu, ST-35 Dubi, ST-36 Zusanli, ST-36 Bis, ST-36 Ter, SP-9 Yinlingquan, SP-10 Xuehai, GB-33 Xiyangguan, GB-34 Yanglingquan, LR-7 Xiguan, LR-8 Ququan, BL-38 Fuxi, BL-39 Weiyang, BL-40 Weizhong, KI-10 Yingu, KI-10 Bis

Channels: *Dumai, Yangqiaomai, Yinqiaomai,* Stomach, Gall Bladder, Kidney, Liver, Spleen

TIBIOTARSAL STRAIN AND PAINFUL FOOT CONDITIONS

Local points: SP-3 Taibai, SP-4 Gongsun, SP-5 Shangqiu, BL-60 Kunlun, BL-61 Pushen, BL-62 Shenmai, BL-63 Jimen, KI-3 Taixi, KI-4 Dazhong, KI-5 Shuiquan, KI-6 Zhaohai, GB-4 Qiuxu, GB-41 Linqi, LR-4 Zhongfeng

Channels: *Yangqiaomai, Yinqiaomai, Dumai,* Gall Bladder, Bladder, Kidney, Liver, Spleen

ACHILLES TENDINITIS

Local points: BL-60 Kunlun, BL-62 Shenmai (see Figure 3.21, page 122), KI-4 Dazhong, EX Genping, EX Quanshengzu, EX Nuxi

Channels: *Yangqiaomai, Yinqiaomai, Dumai,* Gall Bladder, Bladder, Kidney, Liver, Spleen

Nervous System

HEADACHE

Local points: EX-1 Yintang, EX-2 Taiyang, EX-3 Yuyao, EX Erzhong, EX Bitong, EX Neiyingxiang, EX Shangyingxiang, BL-1 Jingming, BL-2 Zanzhu, BL-3 Meichong, BL-4 Quchai, LI-20 Yingxiang, GV-14 Dazhui, VG-15 Yamen, GV-16 Fengfu, BL-10 Tianzhu, BL-1 Dazhu, GB-20 Fengchi, GB-21 Jianjing, TE-15 Tianliao, GV-20 Baihui

Channels: *Chongmai, Dumai, Renmai,* Stomach, Liver, Bladder, Gall Bladder, *Yinweimai, Yangweimai*

MIGRAINE

Local points: On the Gall Bladder Channel, search for points which are painful on their own and during palpation as well as 1 EX-1 Yingdang, EX-2 Taiyang, EX-3 Yuyao, EX Bitong,

EX Neiyingxiang, EX Shangyingxiang, BL-1 Jingming, BL-2 Zanzhu, BL-10 Tianzhu, BL-11 Dazhu, LI-20 Yingxiang, GV-14 Dazhui, GV-15 Yamen, GV-16 Fengfu, GB-20 Fengchi, GB-21 Jianjing, TE-15 Tianliao, GV-20 Baihui

Channels: *Chongmai, Dumai, Renmai*, Stomach, Liver, Bladder, Gall Bladder, *Yinweimai, Yangweimai*

PAIN IN THE CENTRAL AND PERIPHERAL NERVOUS SYSTEMS, NEURITIS

Local points: Use a pointscope to look for the active points that are closest to the seat of the disorder. For neuralgia and neuritis of the head use the same schema as for headache and toothache, for other areas follow the schema for musculoskeletal disorders.

Channels: TMM, *Renmai, Dumai*, Bladder, Stomach

NERVOUS TWITCHING, SHAKING AND TREMORS

Local points: Use a pointscope to look for the active points that are closest to the seat of the disorder. For twitching muscles in the head use the same schema as for headache and toothache.

Channels: *Renmai, Dumai*, Spleen, Lung, Gall Bladder, Liver

ANXIETY AND DEPRESSION, NERVOUS ASTHENIA

Local points: It is not accurate to talk of local points for these disorders, nevertheless use GV-20 Baihui, EX-1 Yingdang, EX-2 Taiyang, KI-3 Taixi, LU-9 Taiyuan, PC-6 Neiguan.

Channels: *Chongmai, Renmai, Dumai*, Stomach, Pericardium, Kidney

Cutaneous system
PRURITUS

Local points: For localised pruritus use a pointscope to look for the active points in the area affected. Also test GV-20 Baihui, BL-40 Weizhong

Channels: *Chongmai, Daimai*, Bladder, Gall Bladder, Stomach, Pericardium, Kidney, Triple Heater

LOCALISED INFLAMMATIONS

Local points: Use a pointscope to look for the active points in the area affected.

Channels: *Renmai, Chongmai*, Lung, Stomach, Kidney

Ears and eyes

ACUTE AND CHRONIC OTALGIA

Local points: SI-17 Tianrong, SI-19 Tinggong, TE-16 Tianyou, TE-17 Yifeng, TE-20 Jiaosun, TE-21 Ermen, GB-2 Tinghui

Channels: *Chongmai*, Kidney, Small Intestine, Pericardium

TINNITUS, VERTIGO AND PRESBYCUSIS

Local points: SI-17 Tianrong, SI-19 Tinggong, TE-16 Tianyou, TR-17 Yifeng, TE-20 Jiaosun, TE-21 Ermen, GB-2 Tinghui

Channels: *Chongmai*, Kidney, Small Intestine, Lung, Pericardium, Gall Bladder, Triple Heater

MIGRAINE AND OPHTHALMIC HEADACHES

Local points: GB-1 Tongziliao, EX-1 Yingdang, EX-2 Taiyang, EX-3 Yuyao, EX Bitong, EX Neiyingxiang, EX Shangyingxiang, BL-1 Jingming, BL-2 Zanzhu, ST-2 Sibai, ST-3 Juliao, BL-3 Meichong, BL-4 Quchai, LI-20 Yingxiang, GV-14 Dazhui, GV-15 Yamen, GV-16 Fengfu, BL-10 Tianzhu, BL-11 Dazhu, GB-20 Fengchi, GB-21 Jianjing, TE-15 Tianliao, GV-20 Baihui, EX-7 Yimen

Channels: *Dumai*, Liver, *Yinweimai, Yinqiaomai*, Gall Bladder

BLEPHARITIS AND BLEPHAROSPASM, MYOPIA, PRESBYOPIA

Local points: GB-1 Tongziliao, EX-1 Yingdang, EX-2 Taiyang, EX-3 Yuyao, EX Bitong, EX Neiyingxiang, EX Shangyingxiang, BL-1 Jingming, BL-2 Zanzhu, ST-2 Sibai, ST-3 Juliao, BL-3 Meichong, BL-4 Quchai, LI-20 Yingxiang, GV-14 Dazhui, GV-15 Yamen, GV-16 Fengfu, BL-10 Tianzhu, BL-11 Dazhu, GB-20 Fengchi, GB-21 Jianjing, TE-15 Tianliao, GV-20 Baihui, EX-7 Yimen

Channels: Liver, Gall Bladder, Kidney, *Chongmai, Renmai*

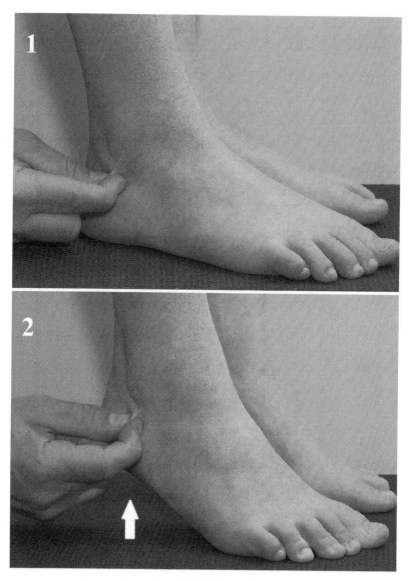

Figure 3.21 The Active Points Test in accordance with the reasoned choice criterion for Achilles tendinitis pain on point BL-62 Shenmai, opening point on the Yangqiaomai channel

The patient is invited to push on to the balls of the feet to highlight the symptom (same case as Figure 3.2, page 73).

Chapter 4

EXPLANATION

4.1 NEUROPHYSIOLOGICAL INTERPRETATION OF THE TEST

The Active Points Test can be interpreted in the light of the 'Gate control system theory', which Melzack and Wall conceived in the 1960s to explain the antalgic effect of the electrical stimulation of the cutis. If it were ever necessary, the Test constitutes clinical confirmation of this theory and in some ways its completion, even though it raises new questions in the relationship between acupoints from the Chinese tradition on the one hand, and modern anatomy and neurophysiology on the other.

According to the theory's authors, the nociceptive stimuli that travel through the pain sensitive pathways along the small-diameter Aδ and C afferent fibres can be inhibited by other stimuli of various kinds (electrical, mechanical, chemical), which are transmitted along the large-diameter Aβ fibres (see Table 2.1, page 42). These two groups of fibres form synapses with the central neurons, sending collaterals to the gelatinous substance of the posterior horn of the spinal cord (Figure 4.1). The current which runs through the large-calibre fibres transmitting therapeutic stimuli has an essentially inhibitory effect on this nervous structure. The 'gate' would therefore be closed to the painful afferents transmitted via the other fibres, due to mutually exclusive competition. The 'gate' can only be concerned with one kind of transmission at a time: nociceptive or tactile (mechanoreceptive–nociceptive).

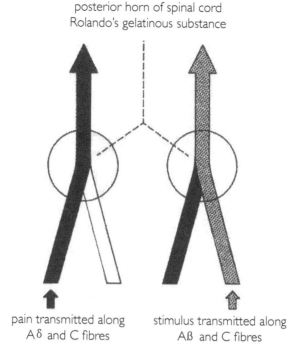

posterior horn of spinal cord
Rolando's gelatinous substance

pain transmitted along
Aδ and C fibres

stimulus transmitted along
Aβ and C fibres

Figure 4.1 Melzack and Wall's Gate control system theory

To quote Hippocrates: 'Of two pains occurring together, not in the same part of the body, the stronger weakens the other.'[35] Originating in the peripheral receptors, the nociceptive signals will travel to the sensory cortex and thus make the individual aware that the body is under a potentially damaging attack. Pinching and superficial puncturing of the skin performed as part of the Test cause pain which, although temporary, is recognised by the sensory cortex as being 'more violent' than any other pain resulting from a medical condition, and so the latter is eclipsed by the former. The Test generates pain sensations similar to those of an animal or plant sting, which trigger strong defence mechanisms because the associative brain, shaped by ancestral experience, immediately identifies them as related to *poisoning, violent immune reaction, lacerations to organs* and consequently to *death*. These sensations instinctively cancel out any other ongoing sensation in order to prepare all systems for the prevention of any organic damage that might threaten survival.

The sensory pathways responsible for transmitting tactile and proprioceptive information stretch through the spinal cord along the lemniscus system. Those responsible for thermal and nociceptive signals travel along the spinothalmic tract. For stimuli applied to the head region, the pathway begins at the level of the medulla oblongata, the pons or the mid-brain where the sensory nuclei of the cranial nerves are situated. Since the Active Points Test may be effective with just one pinch, as we have already seen, and since stimulation of both the mechanoreceptors and the nociceptors is also inevitable with needle puncture, the impulse will be transmitted via either somesthetic method.

From neurophysiology we know that the lemniscus system inhibits the spinothalmic tract on more than one level: from the spinal cord to the thalamus and the sensory cortex. The Active Points Test quickly identifies which spinal or cranial segment is more suitable for inhibiting transmission of the symptom. If the active points are put to the Test, a galaxy of stimuli capable of opposing the patient's disorder on more than one level will be created.

To complete the neurophysiological interpretation, it should be remembered that there is also a synaptic link and a convergence in the somatosensory and viscerosensory conduction pathways. This explains the effect of the Test on symptoms which are not exactly somatic, even though the points being punctured are somesthetic. If the full extent of the sensory pathways is analysed, it can be deduced that there are various ways of interfering with the transmission of the symptom, since each afferent fibre converges and connects with other pathways, ascending and descending, at least at the three levels already mentioned: *spinal cord, thalamus* and *sensory cortex*. The problem is which segment should be chosen in order to counter the symptom, as there is nothing to show that the conduction pathways which are most effective therapeutically originate in the same segment which the symptom in question belongs to.

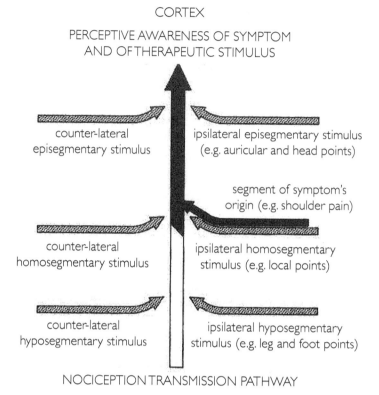

Figure 4.2 Segmental fields (dermatomes) and side on which to choose points and therapy zones after the Active Points Test

The Active Points Test is useful for the diagnosis itself because (Figure 4.2) it allows the practitioner to decide if the optimal level for stimulation is to be found:

- *above the segment where the symptom originated* (episegmentary)
- *at the same level* (homosegmentary)
- *at a lower level* (hyposegmentary).

Furthermore, it helps to decide whether the most effective side for treatment is:

- *the same side as the symptom* (ipsilateral)
- *the opposite side* (counter-lateral).

It is now time to interpret the point activity results (Figure 4.3).

It is easy to explain the existence of local negative points (−), exploration of which causes a worsening of the symptom since, in the presence of a given locoregional symptom such as neck pain or toothache, the sensory fibres of the segment where the diseased zone is situated have a consistently high discharge frequency (from the ordinary receptors, due to the presence of specific inflammatory substances, etc.). Saturation may not be the most suitable term, however, the physiological solutions in which those fibres and receptors are immersed contain without doubt an elevated quantity of pain-generating molecules and mediators. All other stimuli (mechanical, thermal, etc.) will be transformed into painful stimuli, intensifying awareness of the symptom. The famous pain threshold is much lower at this point, and explains why some of the points tested will prove to be *negative*.

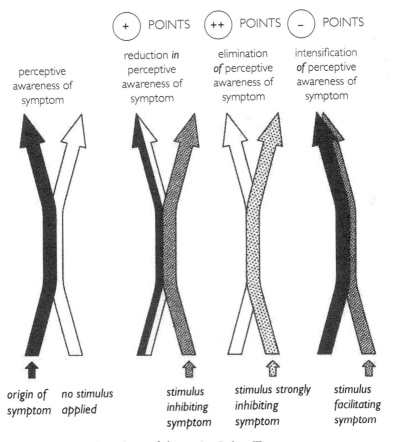

Figure 4.3 Neurophysiology of the Active Points Test

It is more difficult to explain the presence of *negative* points (−) on distal segments and of positive points (+ and + +), both on the same segment and on distal segments. It may be assumed, however, that some segments, together with their relative sensory conduction pathways, have, in a manner of speaking, been 'forgotten', and send few signals to the thalamus and the cortex. Consequently, they are able to compete more easily with the transmission originating in the diseased area and can alter the perception of the symptom. In any case, as stated by Ceccherelli (see page 164):

> We must not forget that it has been proved for years that the therapeutic effect of acupuncture is principally due to the stimulation of the nociceptive mechanoreceptors whose central afferent is connected via the Aδ fibres. These nociceptors have a high threshold and adapt slowly or not at all; this means that the receptor discharges when energy that is potentially damaging to the body is applied, and stops discharging only when the tissue has been destroyed. In the case of the Active Points Test, external stimulation with the tip of a needle, which the patient perceives as a light puncture and a slight pain, is in fact nociceptive stimulation of such receptors. It is, therefore, perfectly understandable for the symptom to show a subjective variation in intensity, albeit brief and fleeting.

4.2 THE QI INTERPRETATION

The Active Points Test may also be explained according to the principles of Traditional Chinese Medicine (TCM), which envisages the channels as being in a state of *fullness* or *emptiness*. The pinching and superficial puncturing with the point of a needle being explored causes defensive *weiqi* energy to enter the channel. Depending on the quantity of *weiqi*, this will result in an attempt to fill or in the complete replenishment of an *empty* channel. This is the reason why points situated on *empty* channels will give *positive* results. Vice versa, if defensive *weiqi* energy enters a full channel, it will become overly full and so the points belonging to it will give *negative* results. Superficial puncturing of channels in a state of equilibrium, which may dilate or contract, will cause the points situated on them to give *indifferent* results.

I do not believe it is coincidence that ancient Chinese doctors categorised some points as *accumulation* points° and others as *hours* points, since they would have observed in them sudden, random or cyclical 'volumetric' manifestations of Qi flow. The patient's involvement in being asked to observe and judge the value of our manoeuvres falls within the sphere of *Shen* which, according to tradition, presides over all forms of consciousness of time and space. It is during the course of the Test between *symptom* → *needle puncture* → *alteration of symptom* that the *Shen* of the *latent awareness of the active point* will show itself.

4.3 *PLACEBO* AND *NOCEBO* EFFECTS

It is useful at this point to mention two factors which can influence the results of the Test. The *placebo* and *nocebo* effects are the two faces of the power of suggestion, and consist of the subjective experience of a 'good' or 'evil' result. This happens during any medical process, whether it is diagnostic or therapeutic.

All of us are susceptible, in varying measure, to the power of suggestion, which brings with it the conviction that whatever has been predicted (even via non-verbal signals) will happen, and causes us to behave in such a way that the prediction will be born out. For example, if we are told that a certain drug is effective in treating the ulcer from which we are suffering, and the person who tells us is someone we consider to be authoritative, competent and 'positive', the probability of our being cured will increase in proportion to our suggestibility, even though the pill being administered actually contains 'nothing'. In reality, this 'nothing' does in fact pass on some information, particularly about the 'positivity' of the person who made the suggestion and the faith we have in that person, and that is no small thing! In medicine, the components of a particular therapy which are neither pharmacological nor neurological are known as the *placebo* effect. The *nocebo* effect is the exact opposite and consists in the appearance of unpleasant and 'negative' symptoms (again, neither

---

o   The Xi-Cleft points.

pharmacological nor neurological) following on from therapy which someone has convinced us will cause sickness.

I do not deny that suggestive factors may play a role during the execution of the Active Points Test, and that the patient might be encouraged to identify the points being explored as positive rather than negative or indifferent. I know of no experiments that have studied a combination of the two opposite types of reaction to suggestion, but I suspect that, given that we are asking the patient a two-fold or three-fold question (with regard to positive, negative and indifferent points), there is much less chance that his or her answers will be influenced by suggestion. I also believe that the Active Points Test may increase the *placebo* effect of therapy, since the fact that we are able to counter the patient's symptoms during the diagnosis itself, through the discovery of positive points, strengthens his or her faith in our diagnostic and therapeutic abilities.

Milani argued that in the field of acupuncture research, because of its many different spheres of action (chemical, physical, psychological...), it is not possible to talk of *placebo points,* even when they are selected in areas which are far from the paths indicated on ancient and modern acupuncture maps.[54] That notwithstanding, attempts to create a technically valid '*sham acupuncture*' still continue. The most recent authors to do this were Streitberger and Kleinhenz,[55] who introduced into acupuncture research a device that acts as a needle without causing the sensation of the skin being punctured.

4.4 PSYCHOLOGICAL IMPLICATIONS

Giovanardi (see page 162) states:

> The thing that struck me most about Dr Marcelli's method is the collaborative relationship that is created between doctor and patient. Asking the patient if the symptom changes during the search for 'positive' points makes him a part of the process and contributes to the effectiveness of acupuncture.

Times have changed and the doctor–patient relationship is becoming ever more equal, with the aim of restoring lost balance. Such balance is greatly sought after by those who practise reflex therapy, especially of a traditional nature, and must be interpreted as belonging not only to the patient, but also to the doctor and society as a whole. Psychoanalysis teaches that unconscious, selfish urges may lie hidden behind every action. In the case of a doctor, behind a façade of willingness to help a sick person he may be hiding *aspirations to dominance over others*, in order to use the patient as a faceless statistic in any one of a thousand *businesses* in the healthcare market.

Doctors must go back to preventing rather than treating. I do not consider it to be a coincidence that my little invention, a rough copy of which had already been traced out by some ancient or modern-day enthusiast of TCM, has been completed by a doctor with as much 'biological' training as 'psychological', and who has chosen the *Natura Medicatrix* as his chief advisor, in harmony with the recent advancements of the last century and millennium.

Rogora, one of the first of my colleagues to whom I had passed on my observations and whose opinion I had sought, told me that my idea reminded him of the method used by the master Quaglia Senta,[47] whose final lessons he had been lucky enough to attend. The master's practice was to manipulate the needles he had stuck into those points considered as 'active' and to immediately ask the patient to tell him how he/she was feeling, after which he extracted those needles that were causing discomfort and left only those which eased the symptom. So, when the patient is asked to concentrate on the sensations caused by the diagnostic movements carried out on his/her body in order to identify the 'active' points, we are in fact increasing his/her awareness of the energy, – it matters little whether we call it *neural current* or Qi – however subtle, which we mean to guide towards giving the patient back his/her health. And there is great value in the fact that it is the patient who directs us onto the right path.

Chapter 5

THERAPY

5.1 THERAPY FOLLOWING THE TEST

Although the procedure for performing the Active Points Test remains the same for all forms of therapy, I would like to offer (to the reader) some suggestions for making the best possible use of its results. Since *negative* points (which make the symptom worse) are rare and *indifferent* points are inactive, I will concentrate principally on the *positive* points (which weaken or neutralise the symptom). Any practitioner may decide in any case to treat the negative and indifferent points as well if they fall within the sphere of those which are considered effective according to the doctrine on which their particular therapy is based. It is worth considering the example of point ST-36 Zusanli, which may be indifferent when tested in relation to gastric pain, but which a traditional acupuncturist may still consider useful for 'strengthening' the *Yang* or the Earth of a patient with the characteristic signs of cold and catarrh (phlegm).

Acupuncture and the cross-shaped pattern
Ignoring the distinction between reflexologists and traditionalists, whoever is competent in the use of needles and has legal permission to practice this therapy will be able to make use of a cross-shaped pattern based on the model inspired by the Sishencong Extra points and modified by me (Figure 5.1). In the area(s) corresponding to the points which showed positive results in the Test, a needle is inserted into the *Centre* in as vertical a position as possible and another four needles are placed at *North*, *South*, *East* and *West* respectively[p] facing obliquely

---

p   Respectively above, below, to the right and to the left of the central point and the practitioner.

towards the *Centre*. The ends of the five needles should be close to one another but should not make contact. The distance between the external points and the central point will vary from a few millimetres where the cutaneous tissue is thin (e.g. on the face and hands), to one or two centimetres where it is thicker (e.g. on the shoulders and gluteal muscles). The needles must stay in position for between 15 minutes to half an hour, and be rotated clockwise and anti-clockwise every four to five minutes. The manipulation will end when *deqi* is achieved and the outcome of the Test is maintained (Figure 5.2). The most important thing during the consultation is to try and follow the lead of the patient, who – as a *sensitive cybernetic organism* – will know if and how his/her symptom changes. I get my bearings by asking him/her if the symptom is eliminated or at least alleviated while the needles are in position. I find out if it has come back by adapting to treatment, in which case manipulation will be required to return to the condition achieved by the insertion of the needles, perhaps by inserting them even deeper or pulling them out, or by repositioning them by a few millimetres.

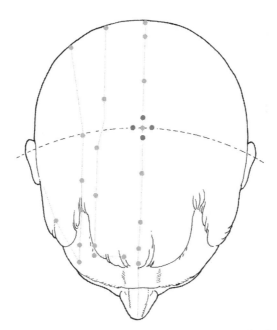

Figure 5.1 Sishencong (Four Intelligence): extra points in the form of a cross around GV-20 Baihui

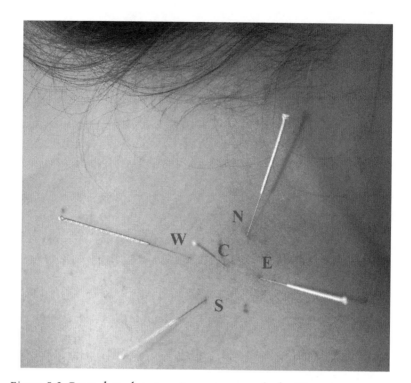

Figure 5.2 Cross-shaped acupuncture pattern used after Test

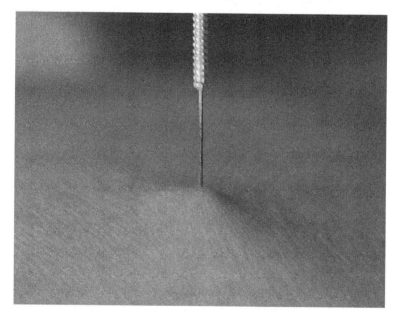

Figure 5.3 The deqi phenomenon

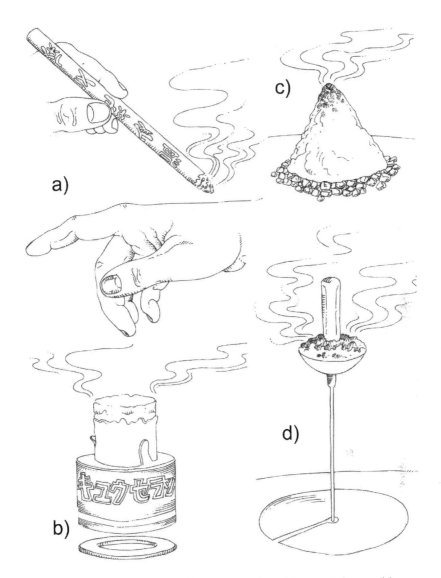

Figure 5.4 Moxibustion with (a) Artemisia cigar (b) ceramic burner (c) moxa wool on salt, garlic and ginger (d) in the hilt of a needle

An aphorism states: 'No result without *deqi*.' I will take this opportunity to explain to those who have little experience of acupuncture that the phenomenon consists of what the French call *saisie de l'energie*, literally 'capturing the energy'. If we have 'got' the point, the skin around the sharp tip of the needle will tighten with such force that it will make extraction difficult (Figure 5.3). The intensity of *deqi* is linked to individual vitality, to the Qi in the channel and to the metal that the needle is made of.[q] If *deqi* is not produced spontaneously, it is advisable to instigate it by patting the end of the needle or rotating or flexing it repeatedly or by heating it. I have always managed to find *deqi* in points that showed positive results during the Test, and this is a further sign of its usefulness in the practice of acupuncture. Moxibustion with moxa-cigars or a heated needle may also be used on positive points (Figure 5.4). The effect of moxa on positive points lasts longer than the effect of a needle, since first degree burns caused by this method generate a slight persistent burning sensation that prolongs the stimulation of the Test.

Blisters from second degree burns, which are rare but possible when using a moxa-cigar, especially where there is reduced sensitivity to pain, and above all third degree necroses are generally to be avoided. They may be useful only in chronic and rebellious cases, and should be kept to a minimum by using the smallest possible quantities of moxa. Another useful technique is to apply suction cups to *positive* points, which are as effective for the Test as pinching or needling in cases of blood stagnation. This is also true of bloodletting performed with a triangular needle on dilated capillaries found next to or near *positive* points. I am sure that one of the reasons that mesotherapy is so effective in the treatment of pain can be traced back to the extensive bleeding induced by *nappage* (see below). In my opinion, this is not the place to linger over the age-old question of the dispelling, reinforcing and harmonising effects of the techniques described, as they only make sense in a discussion purely about TCM.[r] In my experience, only

---

q   Before the introduction of single use needles and the ever more frequent allergies to nickel, it was common practice at least in the French school to choose needles of gold alloy (and nickel) for toning, and needles of silver alloy for dispersion.

r   Moxibustion is generally considered to be reinforcing, while the application of suction cups and bleeding are thought to have a dispelling effect. The effect of moxa is considered to be dispelling if it is applied to the stem of a needle that has already been inserted. The question is considered to be as controversial by the traditional school of thought as it is by contemporary authors. Through arduous application during the Test, I have noticed that points which respond a few of the cases that were sensitive to the Test did not respond to needle stimulation (*relative non-responders*). In two of these, the symptom was essential neuralgia of the trigeminal nerve [*sic!*]. After a few acupuncture sittings, during which the benefit lasted a few minutes after the extraction of the needles, the symptom gave in to intradermal injections of 0.1 ml of the cocktail *Procaine 2% 1 ml, Clorproetazine*[s] *1 vial, physiological solution 4 ml* into each the active point. This is a classic mesotherapy cocktail for articular pain.

Auricular puncture

This will almost seem to be a continuation of the above discussion about moxa and bleeding. With the permission of the publisher, I will quote a few passages by Paul Nogier, who devised the method, which refer to 'evidence of practices in which a rudimentary form of auricular therapy can be picked out'.[56]

> In actual fact, the origins of these practices are lost in the mists of time. Does the Tradition come from Egypt, Persia or China? No-one will ever know for sure. On the other hand, we do know that the Egyptians used the stimulation of a few points on the auricle to alleviate certain pains. Hippocrates refers to healing impotence by inducing small amounts of bleeding on the ear. Throughout the centuries, documents have been found which talk about similar treatments for curing various illnesses.
>
> In 1637, a Portuguese doctor called Zacutus Lusitanus described the usefulness of cauterising the ear in the treatment of sciatic nerve neuralgia.
>
> In 1717 in a written work entitled: 'De aura humana tractatus', Valsalva identifies on pages 11 and 12, paragraph 15, the area of the auricle which would be burned to treat bad toothache. In

---

positively to needles do so also to moxa, and this is explained by the notion that the stimuli induced by both puncturing and heating over and above a certain threshold are nociceptive and follow the same nervous conduction pathway, despite activating two separate receptors.

s   Clorproetazine is a neuroleptic myorelaxant that acts on the motor end plate, which was used in anaesthetic premedication until ten years ago, but is no longer available today (Neuriplege®). It can be replaced with vitamin B12, vitamin C, or with bidistilled water, which are just as painful when injected.

1810, a doctor from Parma, Professor Ignazio Colla, described the case of a man who, after being stung by a bee on the ear at the level of the antihelix, was temporarily unable to walk. In the same publication, he mentions cases of retroauricular cauterisation, successfully carried out on his advice by a fellow surgeon, Dr Lecconi, for the treatment of sciatic nerve pain. In 1850, Dr Rülker from Cincinnati referred to a good outcome in a case of sciatica obtained by cauterising the helix. Following this, in the same year in a series of observations and documents, Dr Lucciani di Bastia recommended the cauterisation of the helix as a radical treatment for sciatica. In the same period, Professor Malgaigne from the Saint Louis Hospital pointed out in his clinical bulletin the rather surprising results obtained with this technique. Between 1850 and 1857, numerous publications talking about this treatment and expressing the amazement of the physicians of the time came out in France and a real infatuation for this method caught on, although it was rather short-lived due to the fact that it was not supported by any scientific basis. In spite of everything, a century later around 1951, doctors from the area around Lyon found they were being consulted by a few patients with strange cauterisations on the auricle, who claimed they had been cured of sciatic neuralgia thanks to this kind of operation.[t]

As striking today as they are unfeasible, even though we should *never say never,* these cauterisations show that the treatment of *the active points* in auricular puncture is nothing new. Needling will be performed with auricular puncture needles, possibly using semi-permanent ones or fixing vaccaria seeds to the ear with plasters. It is advisable to keep an auricular map close by the couch (examination bed), so that it may be consulted during the sitting. Here are depicted both an iconographic map showing drawings of the organs to help the beginner identify zones and points to be subjected to the Test and to therapy (Figure 5.5), and a centrographic map with points and legend (Figure 5.6 and Table 5.1). Practice will gradually bring familiarity with most of the

---

[t]   The cicatricial results of an identical practice were also observed by me in the 1980s in patients from the countryside near Cremona, carried out as treatment for sciatica by 'a local healer of gypsy origin'.

important points. Beginners and those who are not legally permitted to use needles may avail themselves of a specific massager or an electrical stimulator. For further tips, they should consult the works of Romoli and other entries in the endnotes section.

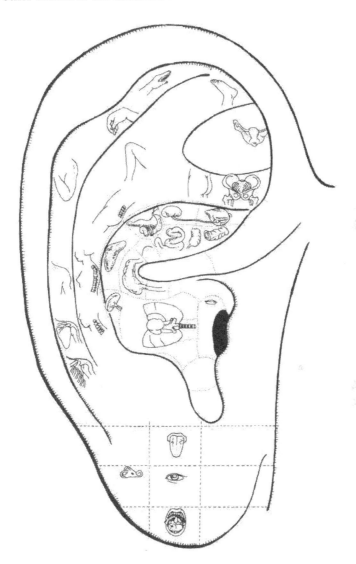

Figure 5.5 Iconographic auricular puncture map

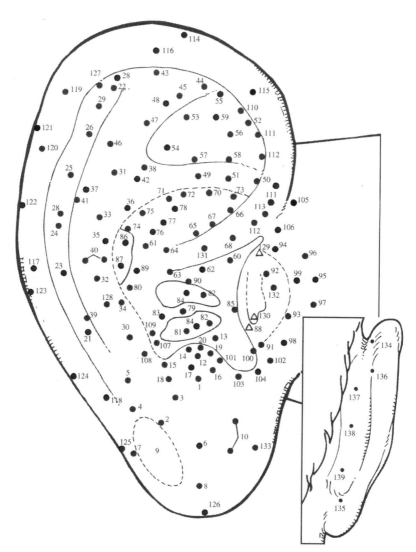

Figure 5.6 Centrographic auricular puncture map
Lateral and medial face (bottom right corner) of the auricle. The points marked
by a triangle are covered by the tragus. Legend in Table 5.1.

TABLE 5.1 LEGEND FOR FIGURE 5.6

Lateral face

1) Lower palate
2) Upper palate
3) Tongue
4) Maxilla
5) Mandible
6) Eye
7) Ear
8) Tonsil
9) Cheek
10) Analgesic point for dental extraction
11) Parotid gland
12) Asthma
13) Testicle
14) Cerebral point
15) Occiput
16) Forehead
17) Great *Yang*
18) Cranial Vertex
19) Subcutis
20) Stimulating point
21) Clavicle
22) Finger
23) Shoulder joint
24) Shoulder
25) Elbow
26) Wrist
27) Nephritis point
28) Appendix point
29) Urticaria point
30) Cervical vertebrae
31) Sacral vertebrae
32) Thoracic vertebrae
33) Lumbar vertebrae

34) Neck
35) Thorax
36) Abdomen
37) External abdominal wall
38) Colon point
39) Thyroid
40) Breast
41) Appendicular abdominal point
42) Lumbalgia point
43) Big toe
44) 5th toe
45) Ankle
46) Knee
47) Hip
48) Knee joint
49) Coccyx
50) Sympathetic nervous system
51) Sciatic nerve point
52) Uterus-prostate
53) Shenmen sedation
54) Pelvic excavation
55) Hypotensive point
56) Asthma point
57) Coxofemoral joint
58) Constipation point
59) Hepatitis point
60) Mouth
61) Stomach
62) Oesophagus
63) Cardia
64) Duodenum
65) Small intestine
66) Large intestine
67) Appendix

68) Diaphram
69) Centre of the ear
70) Bladder
71) Kidney
72) Ureter
73) Prostate
74) Liver
75) Pancreas
76) Pancreatitis point
77) Ascites point
78) Drunkeness point
79) Heart
80) Spleen
81) Lung
82) Bronchial tube
83) Tuberculosis point
84) Bronchiectasis
85) Trachea
86) Cirrhosis zone
87) Hepatomegaly zone
88) Triple heater
89) Hepatitis zone
90) New eye point
91) Upper nose point
92) Throat
93) Corticoadrenale point
95) Wings of the nose
96) Thirst point
97) Hunger point
98) Hypertensive point
99) Eustachian tube
100) Endocrine point
101) Ovary
102) Eye 1
103) Eye 2
104) Hypertensive point 2

105) External ear

106) Cardiac point

107) Cerebral trunk

108) Soft palate

109) Toothache point

110) External genitals

111) Urethra

112) Rectum

113) Anus

114) Apex of the ear

115) Punto of blindness

116) Tonsil 1

117) Tonsil 2

118) Tonsil 3

119) Liver 1

120) Liver 2

121) Helix point 1

122) Helix point 2

123) Helix point 3

124) Helix point 4

125) Helix point 5

126) Helix point 6

127) Small occipital nerve

128) Thyroid

129) Lower abdomen

130) Upper abdomen

131) Deaf and dumb point

132) General nervous system

133) Neurasthenia

Medial face

134) Spinal cord 1

135) Spinal cord 2

136) Hypotensive point

137) Lumbosacral column

138) Thoracic and lumbar column

139) Cervical and thoracic column

Mesotherapy

The effectiveness of mesotherapy can be traced back to the five action mechanisms.[27] The first is *suggestion*, which is common to all therapies in varying degree. The second is *puncture*, shared by all methodologies involving needling and multiple injections. The third is *bleeding*, which has not been greatly emphasised by the big names in mesotherapy, perhaps because of the ban on bloodletting in modern medicine.[u] The fourth is *anaesthetic*. The fifth and final one relates to the specific properties of the other *drugs* present in the cocktails. Despite being a drug, anaesthetic is considered to be a therapeutic factor in its own right insofar as it is common in neural therapy and is an indispensable component of the cocktails. Mesotherapeutic treatment of points which show positive results to the Test will follow the cross-shaped pattern indicated for acupuncture. In lieu of needles, microinjections of 0.2 ml of the cocktail, prepared previously, will be administered in each of the five points: *Centre, North, South, East* and *West*, taking care to direct the needle towards the central point (Figure 5.7). The microinjections will be followed by *nappage* (see Figure 2.1, page 35), with a distance between the punctures of 1–3 mm, striking the area already explored during the search for points and concentrating most of the punctures on the point at the centre. If there is no clear

---

u   It should be pointed out, however, that the use of leeches has made a come-
     back in the field of cosmetic surgery and articular pain.

perception of the symptom, treatment will proceed according to the classic method: microinjections and *nappage* in the affected areas indicated by the patient and by a clinical examination performed manually and with instruments. After mesotherapy, treatment can be performed with acupuncture needles using the cross-shaped pattern.

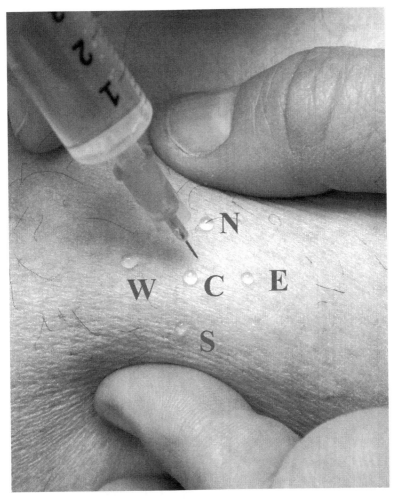

Figure 5.7 Mesotherapy performed on the active point after the Test, microinjections administered in the form of a cross

Neural therapy

As already stated, neural therapy consists of a superficial or deep injection of the anaesthetic *procaine*, which is administered in a concentration of 1% or 2%, and in doses of 10 ml or 5 ml respectively per sitting, hence not in the modest quantities used in mesotherapy. If the Test is interpreted only according to the Gate control theory, then neural therapy must be directed exclusively at negative points. Nevertheless, I have been able to ascertain that injections of anaesthetic (procaine or lidocaine) in positive points are as effective as inserting a needle in chronic cases, while the effect *may* be stronger in acute cases but is certainly more enduring. The injection of anaesthetic is, in my opinion, an indispensable tool for achieving an effective treatment for the few points which give *negative* results to the Test, especially if treatment of *positive* points has produced unsatisfactory results.

Due consideration must be given to the fact that it is difficult to establish the exact place of anaesthetic in the neurophysiological interpretation of the Test, because the Gate control theory does not contemplate the possibility that neutralising cutaneous afferents can act to inhibit pain as much as stimulating them. The difficulty derives from the fact that, unlike accidental puncture, local anaesthetic practically does not exist in nature, although it is in some ways similar to a cold compress, often used to treat painful conditions and particularly useful for acute traumas of the locomotive system.

Manual techniques

Massotherapists, like practitioners of shiatsu and tuina, physiotherapists, chiropractors, experts in Rolfing or connective tissue massage, will be able to manipulate *positive* points using the standard procedure of their specialty. There would certainly be no conflict if they were to give greater attention to points resulting *positive* to the Test than to those which they would usually treat, just as there would be no conflict in using the *pincé roulé* to improve circulation and break the fibrous bonds which bind the *positive* points to certain areas and to the subcutis. *Positive* points can be treated using the cross-shaped pattern described below, obviously through manual stimulation.

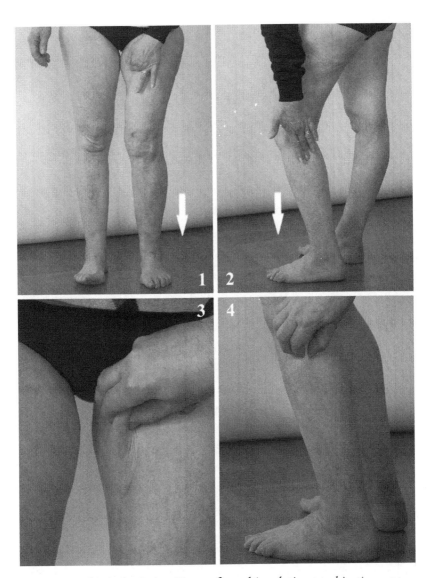

Figure 5.8 The Active Points Test performed in relation to a kinetic symptom (sciatica)

The patient communicates that: 'When I put my weight on my left foot it hurts (1) here, and (2) here. (3) and (4) Execution of the Test on the most painful local points – while the patient performs the movement which triggers the pain – corresponding to the extra points Jiaoling (Liver Channel) and Zuyicong (Gall Bladder Channel).

5.2 IN SUMMARY

I have compared the Active Points Test to the antibiogram, and it can rightly be said that the choice of an antibiotic made in accordance with the results of an antibiogram has a favourable influence on therapy. Nevertheless, just as the antibiogram gives no indication as to the dose of the specific antibiotic, or to how and for how long it should be administered, so the Active Points Test gives no information as to how therapy on the active points should be carried out. The only clear indication seems to be to stimulate the *positive* points. How to do this is of little importance. The important thing is that it works, and that the effect lasts as long as possible. Experience will suggest the most opportune method. Here are the stages I generally use in mine:

1. In the first two sittings, I only treat the *positive* points with classic acupuncture needles using the cross-shaped pattern described above. If these are effective and there is steady improvement, I continue with the treatment until the problem is cured. However, I never have more than 4–5 sittings, carried out once or twice a week or even daily depending on the severity of the symptom.

2. If at the first sitting, or at most the second, the points prove to be ineffective, despite their obvious positivity (the *relative non-responders*), I move on to pharmacological mesotherapy, still using the cross-shaped pattern.

3. If even that is not enough, I administer superficial and deep anaesthetic to the active points using the same method as described for the previous point but using only a 2% procaine solution.[v]

Acupuncture was not effective only in the cases of trigeminal neuralgia mentioned earlier, whose symptoms were later alleviated through injection, and in the few cases of arthritic pain with serious joint degeneration, which I decided to treat with mesotherapy or

---

v   Practitioners of mesotherapy and neural therapy are strongly advised to carry out a tolerance test before every sitting and with the same cocktail. This is performed by putting a small drop of the product on the skin of the inside of the forearm, then passing through it with the needle without putting any pressure on the pump of the syringe and avoiding the vessels. Itching, the appearance of spontaneous papules, broken capillaries, horripilation, perspiration, alterations in cardiac rhythm or a general feeling of malaise will lead to the suspension of the operation.

neural therapy after realising that, although stimulation worked, its effectiveness was short-lived. It was incumbent on me not to deprive the patient of immediate, lasting relief from the symptom, and to limit the cost of treatment. If I evaluate my protocol according to TCM, I think that stimulation with needles or drugs is preferable in *cold* subjects, the depressed and asthenic suffering from numb pain (the *Yin* ones of the Tradition), while anaesthetic injections are more indicated in *warm* subjects, the euphoric and hyperstenic suffering from acute pain (the *Yang* ones of tradition).

5.3 CLINICAL CASES

The results of the Active Points Test and of the therapy that followed it in some cases from clinical practice will now be shown. The first three refer to regional affections, while the other two relate to general affections. In order to make it easy to understand, I have chosen to show only cases where I could not find negative points and where therapy was carried out using only acupuncture needles and not in conjunction with injections and other reflex techniques.

WALTER A.

Aged 38, a building contractor who also drives an excavator. He had been suffering for a year from bilateral epicondylitis, which at that time was more painful in the right elbow. He had had surgery on the left elbow one month prior to consulting me.

Case history

Appendectomy, fracture to the right radius, operation to reduce a fracture to the left tibia and fibula, gastroduodenal ulcer since age 25 affected by seasonal changes, with worsening of condition in spring and autumn (cimetidine when necessary).

Therapy and results

CV-12 Zhongwan (on which were found lipoma-like formations of a few centimetres in diameter) and BL-62 Shenmai bilaterally were strongly positive, BL-60 Kunlun bilaterally and KI-6 Zhaohai were positive, as was the auricular elbow point bilaterally. Pain and functional limitation disappeared after six weekly sittings. Pain disappeared when pressure applied to tested points.

GIOVANNI

Aged 46, builder. He had been suffering for two months from continuous pain and functional limitation to the right shoulder which set in after lifting an excessively heavy weight.

Case history

Appendectomy, fracture of the internal right malleolus following a road accident, chronic bronchitis caused by smoking (constant use of mucolytic agents for insistent chronic cough), eczema occurring during the summer months on the back of the hands with small blisters and honey-like secretions.

Therapy and results

LU1-Zhongfu, LU2-Yumen and BL-62 Shenmai on the right side only, were positive. At the second sitting the pain was no longer continuous but set in only during arm abduction, with a noticeable reduction in functional weakness. Point BL-62 Shenmai was no longer positive, LU1-Zhongfu and LU2-Yumen were slightly positive. Points LR-2 Xiangjian and LV-3 Taichong were strongly positive. At the third sitting, pain and functional weakness both disappeared. The patient complained of thoracic dorsalgia in the median line. GV-14 Dazhui and GB-21 Jianjing, TE-15 Tianliao and SI-3 Houxi, all on the right side, were positive during the Test. All symptoms disappeared at the fourth weekly sitting.

RENATO

Aged 46, textile worker. He had been suffering from acute pain in the neck and right shoulder with irradiation at the wrist for a few days (the first half of March). Mobility in the upper limbs and neck was very limited. No painful points during palpation. No clinical or instrumental investigation.

Case history

The only relevant fact was a gastroduodenal ulcer 20 years previously, treated through diet, antacids and receptor-antagonists. No further digestive disorders experienced following this treatment.

Therapy and results

Being a case of acute pain, I immediately analysed the most active points on the Extraordinary Channels whose upper passages cross the area of the neck and shoulder: the *Yang* and *Yin* Vessels of the ankle, discovering that point BL-62 Shenmai gave strongly positive results to the Test. Because the case history showed previous occurrence of a gastric condition, I explored the Stomach Channel and discovered that point ST-41 Jiexi was positive during the Test (still in relation to the patient's acute pain). Striking and immediate disappearance of symptoms at the end of the one and only sitting carried out immediately after the examination.

GABRIELLA

Aged 45, school teacher. She had been suffering for ten years from erythematous lesions on her eyelids (betamethasone or fluocortolone ointment applied every evening), intense itching, redness and swelling extending to the zygomatic region. Periodic appearance of scaly, intensely itchy eczema behind the auricle and also intense pruritus in the ear passage. She wanted to free herself of her dependence on drugs, especially cortisone treatments, suspension of which would, however, aggravate the dermatological picture.

Case history

At age 20, operation to reduce a fracture to the right femur sustained in a road accident, at age 35 serious depression treated with psychopharmaceuticals (fluvoxamine and etizolam, which she was still taking in reduced doses) and psychotherapy, persistent oxyuriasis since adulthood, current insomnia (previously treated with flunitrazepan and then with zolpidem before bedtime), headaches brought on by foods such as chocolate, mayonnaise, fried food, butter and fatty cheese. She had been taking sexual hormones for a year (ethinylestradiol / desogestrel) to treat delays in her menstrual cycle.

Therapy and results

I asked the patient to avoid applying the cortisone cream for one evening and to come and see me the next day. The lesions were very ugly to look at, extremely red, swollen and itchy. Point GB-43 Xiaxi gave strongly positive results to the Test in relation to the pruritus. I asked her to go back to using the ointment, but to reduce its concentration by half by mixing it in equal proportions with a neutral cream. At the next sitting a week later, the lesions showed noticeable improvement, she had not had any more headaches and even her insomnia had improved. There was strong pruritus on the head and dandruff. She suffered from such problems periodically and used an anti-dandruff shampoo. A stye had appeared on her upper right eyelid. At the third sitting a week later, point GB-43 Xiaxi was still strongly positive. At the fourth sitting, everything had improved and the patient was using the cortisone cream at half its original concentration just once a week. She now had, however, a stomach ache with feeling of gastric heaviness from which she had previously suffered in the past (treated with antacids). GB-43 Xiaxi, GB-1 Tongziliao and TE-23 Sizhukong were positive in relation to the itching from the eczema on the eyelid, GB-43 Xiaxi and LR-3 Taichong were positive in relation to the gastralgia. After a week, all the dermatological lesions had disappeared (she had stopped using the cortisone ointment), as had the stomach ache. The insomnia had also gone (use of hypnotic drugs suspended). Treatment concluded after four sittings.

ANGELO

Aged 38, a foreman working in the metal alloy die-casting industry. He was suffering from a recurring frontal headache and a sensation of blockage in the digestive system, with belching, a bitter taste in the mouth, alterations in his sense of balance, nausea and slight problems with his sight which was tired and blurred. Sleep was unsatisfactory. These problems would last for approximately a week to ten days, but at other times his health was just about normal, except for diffuse lumbar pain which became more intense with changes in the weather conditions.

Case history

Nothing in particular, except for the detection by X-ray of long radius left-convex thoracic scoliosis and the calcification of a right paravertebral lymph node. A gastroscopy performed approximately one year earlier showed diffuse gastropathy with slight erosion of the duodenal bulb. In the same period, a Holter monitor recorded numerous benign extrasystoles.

Therapy and results

At the first sitting a week after the consultation, the patient presented complaining of lumbalgia. Palpation of the abdomen revealed pain in the epigastric and mesogastric region. I invited him to exert pressure on the painful areas and at the same time to indicate to me which of the points I was testing brought about an improvement in the symptom. SI-3 Houxi on the right (opening point of the Governing

Vessel), CV-15 Jiuwei, CV-12 Zhongwan and GB-14 Yangbai, in the area where his headache was localised, were all strongly positive. GV-3 Yangyaoguan, BL-60 Kunlun and BL-62 Shenmai on the left only were all positive for the lumbar pain. At the second sitting a week later, the patient reported that the lumbar and gastric pains had disappeared and that there had been improvement in his digestion and related symptoms. Palpation of the epigastric and mesogastric region still caused pain and only points CV-15 Jiuwei and CV-12 Zhongwan gave positive results. At the third sitting, the patient reported that he was completely healthy and examination by pressing hard on the abdomen provided objective proof that the gastric pain had disappeared.

5.4 DISCUSSION AND CONCLUSIONS

An analysis of the cases described shows how the points giving positive results to the Active Points Test are always found on energy passages that have already been disturbed in some way, as in the case of Giovanni's chronic cough and Gabriella's digestive disorders. In the first case, there was an energy imbalance in the Lung Channel which affected the way the shoulder functioned. In the second case, the eczema was simply one of the manifestations of a disturbance in the Gall Bladder Channel, as were the insomnia (the channel's energy peak is between 23:00 and 1:00) and the headache which set in after the consumption of fatty foods. Here, the medical case history also reported a fracture of the femur, a sign perhaps of premature weakening or a predisposing physical cause of the disturbance in the Channel (blind acupuncture?). In the case of the last patient, Angelo, it was obvious that the pre-existing cause of the stomach condition was the vertebral scoliosis. And it was precisely SI-3 Houxi, the opening point of the *Dumai* Extraordinary Channel, which is the Governing Vessel of the vertebral column, that tested positive in relation to the patient's symptoms.

The case of Renato deserves special attention. In acute cases such as this the Test is invaluable since it almost always leads to the discovery of strongly positive points and allows the ongoing problems to be dealt with in a short period of time. As a matter of fact, channels related to an acute disease show clear alterations in energy. This case demonstrates the importance of using the Test to experiment with the seasonal reducing and reinforcing points in relation to acute diseases and flare-ups. This is yet another empirical demonstration of the truth of the Chinese doctrine which states that some points possess more seasonal energy than others. Point ST-41 Jiexi is in fact the *fire point* of the Stomach Channel and puncturing it in spring disperses *wood* energy, a characteristic of this season, in accordance with the law of the five elements.

Chapter 6
PERSPECTIVES

6.1 USE OF THE TEST IN BORDERLINE CASES

Many diseases present in an insidious way, giving the patient a general feeling of malaise without a clear perception of it. Neurologically, this corresponds to an imprecise localisation of the symptom somewhere on the body, ineffectively projected onto the cerebral cortex which is assigned to receiving and processing sensory afferents.

The Active Points Test can be carried out even when there is no clear perception of the symptom. The difficulty resides in stimulating the patient's sensitivity and ability to make observations. If we decide to subject a patient suffering from hypochromic anaemia to acupuncture, we will naturally choose from those points which are known to increase the number of red blood cells, or which 'invigorate the blood', like points ST-36 Zusanli and SP-10 Xuehai. Generally speaking, the active points for hypochromic anaemia (a form of blood deficiency) are those that, whether directly or indirectly, increase the number of red blood cells. These points take effect at a slower rate than those which alleviate pain in joints, since their ultimate target is not the nervous system. During testing in relation to an easily localised symptom such as epicondylitis, the information transmitted to the patient's consciousness telling him or her that a point is positive travels at the conduction speed of the nerve fibres, which is never less than 5–10 m/s. The patient receives the stimulus in a few hundredths of a second and his or her response arrives after a few seconds, which is the time needed to process the effect of the stimulus from the symptom.

Conversely, pinching or contact with a needle on a point acting on the stomach to increase the absorption of iron, or on the bone marrow to boost the production of red blood cells, or on the liver and spleen in order to slow down damage, takes effect at a much slower rate, in the order of hours or days. With these kinds of diseases, therefore, it is difficult if not impossible for the patient to communicate how he or she is feeling immediately after the Test. I have used the Test in relation to diseases such as hypochromic anaemia and endogenous depression, with good results. I asked the patients to concentrate intensely so as to perceive even the slightest difference in the symptom after the needle made contact with the points (this is the most effective method). In the anaemia cases, I asked the patients to pay attention to any changes in their overall strength, to any feelings of increase in muscle strength. In the cases of endogenous depression, I tried to relate the Test to ideation and imagination, as well as to positive feelings since, as every traditional acupuncturist knows, psychic forces are also controlled by acupoints.

6.2 SELF-ADMINISTRATION

Self-administration of the Active Points Test is to be applied in cases where symptoms do not occur on a continuous basis, or in those where the circumstances are such as to make its execution by the practitioner impossible. That is to say for patients who live a long way from their usual doctor, who are suffering from symptoms which only set in at night or during the weekend (weekend headache), during wet weather or when the north wind is blowing, or which recur on an irregular basis. In such cases, the patient will be asked to administer the Test when the symptoms appear, before taking any medication, even herbal or homeopathic. I give drawings of the points that should be tested when the symptom is ongoing, with orders to pinch the skin in accordance with the *pincé roulé* method, to those of my patients whom I consider capable of administering the Test by themselves. For older or less 'practical' patients, I mark their bodies with a skin marker at the points which, according to my diagnosis, are more likely to be active. The mark left by a common felt-tip pen will only last a few days, so it is important to remind the patient to redraw it so as not to lose the position of the acupoint.

Instructions for execution of the Test can also be entrusted to a close relative if points on the back or the ear have to be examined. In any case, the practitioner will have the results communicated to him or her so that he or she will be able to carry out therapy along the lines of the invaluable information given to him/her.

6.3 TOWARDS A MORE RATIONAL THERAPY

The Active Points Test makes acupuncture more rational, because its practices are subjected to a veracity test. Let's take again the example of desensitisation therapy using specific allergens in the field of allergy prevention, which is logically indicated only after the execution of a Radioallergosorbent test (RAST) or other test which will objectively demonstrate the occurrence in the body of a reaction to a given allergen. If, then, the appearance in spring of rhinorrhea with conjunctivitis, which gets worse on clear, windy days, and the presence of poplars in the vicinity of the patient's house, are sufficient elements to arouse suspicion of a seasonal allergy and to establish a specific symptomatic treatment, whether natural or chemical, they are not sufficient to diagnose *an allergy to poplar pollen* and undertake a specific therapy of desensitisation using dilutions of that particular allergen. But neither would it be right to prescribe antihistamines without the certainty of an actual reaction to histamine in the body. Nevertheless, because antihistamines are relatively innocuous, they are often prescribed despite the lack of any evidence in advance (other than clinical suspicion) that they are necessary.

Another example which has already been mentioned is the antibiogram, an *in vitro* test which controls therapy with antibiotics. Whenever possible, antibiotics should be administered on the basis of a diagnostic test – culture plus antibiogram – which indicates whether a germ really is present and which molecules it is most sensitive to. However, they are often used in a superficial way. This has led to their indiscriminate use, more along the lines of a consumer model than a scientific one, which over time has weakened their therapeutic effectiveness, giving rise to numerous kinds of resistant micro-organisms. The equivalent of this conduct in the field of acupuncture is the overuse of points which have a strong general effect and the neglect of those which are 'causal'.

By making it easier to diagnose effective points, the Active Points Test makes any traditional or reflex methodology's therapy more rational, regardless of whether diagnostic models belonging to modern neurology are being used or whether the patient is being examined according to the rules of Traditional Chinese Medicine (TCM). To illustrate this, I need to refer to an important clinical case.

When I was presenting the Test to my colleagues from the Associazione Medici Agopuntori Bolognesi, at the end of the conference I proposed to give a practical demonstration. The volunteer was a fellow physiatrist who had been suffering for two weeks from cervicalgia with intense pain when flexing and turning the head, with significant limitation in his range of movements on both sides of the neck. He had undergone manipulation of the rachis and mesotherapy with non-steroidal anti-inflammatory drugs (NSAIDs), both without results.

The only detail worthy of note revealed in the case history was that he had been suffering from seasonal rhinitis brought on by allergy for two years. During the Test, SI-3 Houxi on the right was mildly positive and GV-26 Renzhong was strongly positive. The Huatuojiaji between C4 and C5 on the left were positive, as was GB-21 Jianjing on the left shoulder, while the counter-laterals were negative. GV-14 Dazhui was indifferent. EX-1 Yingdang was also positive. On the Lung Channel, tested in relation to the seasonal rhinitis, LU-10 Yuji, spring dispersion point of the Lung Channel, was positive (it was in fact a spring evening). I asked my other fellow traditional acupuncturists to indicate to me a point which, according to the law of the five elements, should have been negative and should have aggravated the neck symptom. SP-3 Taibai was suggested by one of them, but the result of the Test was indifferent. Another colleague pointed out that TCM traces a stiff neck back to the Liver-Gall Bladder lodge and suggested that I test LR-3 Taichong. Well, that point proved to be *the most active of all* tested points, as well as being quite painful when I pressed on it with my index finger while trying to locate it. My colleague's problem was relieved almost completely during the demonstration by the insertion of needles into the *positive* points. When I telephoned him a few days later, he told me that just by puncturing point LR-3 Taichong again the afternoon following the conference, the results obtained the previous evening had been stabilised.

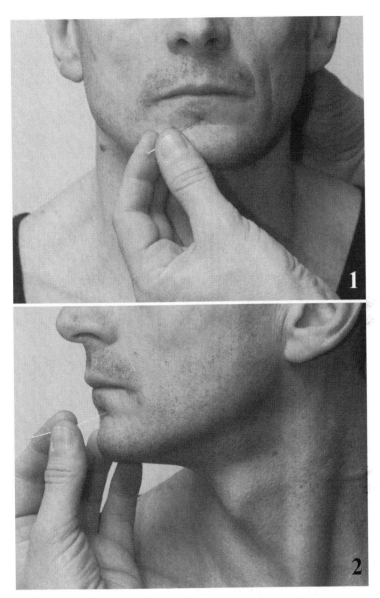

Figure 6.1 The Active Points Test performed by a needle (Needle Contact Test) in a kinetic symptom: acute neck sprain with pain and movement block
The needle is only put in contact with (1) CV-24 Chengjiang point, while asking the patient to do the movement (2) provoking or exalting the symptom, in this case the head rotation to right, and to refer any change in pain perception and rotation limitation.

Chapter 7

EXPERT OPINIONS

7.1 IN ORDER OF ARRIVAL

In this chapter are quoted the opinions of a few of my colleagues given when the first edition of the book was published. I am happy that I belong to a group of doctors who have 'actively' humble, open minds, since almost all of those whom I approached were willing to 'verify' my claims and to 'experiment' with the Active Points Test on their own patients.

Although I have chosen the names on the basis of my present or past association with them, I apologise to anyone – Italian or otherwise – who may be unhappy that they were not consulted. I renew my thanks to those who responded.

Carlo Di Stanislao

An eclectic acupuncturist, dermatologist and author of numerous publications of value in the field of acupuncture. He was a co-editor of the Italian edition of Meck Manual and is a teacher at the Italo-Chinese school of acupuncture. Here is his learned opinion:

> Men consider what they know and do not notice that knowledge begins only when, on the basis of what is well-known, one considers what is not known.
>
> (Zhuangzi: 369–286 a. C.)

Three times in my life have I felt really embarrassed, that is to say self-conscious, worried, confused, overcome by my inability to react quickly and skilfully.

The first time was while reading, as an adolescent, the erotic verse of Gibran *(Locked in a violent embrace. The mystery of the womb that you can penetrate. You penetrate me, you are powerful, you are happy, but after this each moment will be mine).* The second time was a few years ago, facing my father, who was gravely ill, and being unable to communicate my affection for him about which I had kept silent for too long. And now, after reading *The Active Points Test*, I am embarrassed by the unpretentious intelligence of the text, the fresh clarity of the concepts, the brevity and rigorousness of the chapters, the clear and never dogmatic language, and the virginal transparency of the content. Using a speculative methodology, the work analyses in depth and interprets a thousand-year-old science whose archetypes and assumptions have eluded us since time immemorial.

To have realised that the 'kinesiologic' key could act as a guide to diagnosis and reflex treatment is both banal and extraordinary: a reality within the reach of all but missed by everyone else.

Let's be clear, Marcelli's work cannot be called strictly phenomenological, since it is not a simple and aesthetic description of phenomena as they present themselves in an experience: rather it is a Hegelian or Husserlian work: a method (or path in the Conradian sense of the word) along which the reader is able to achieve (progressively) a kind of absolute self-consciousness. In other words, the subject develops like phenoplastic condensation a chemical reaction, overcoming empirical or overly individual conclusions (through objective data), to arrive at 'different' and 'palpable' interpretations of the truth of Chinese acupuncture.

However, my practical tests (repeated more than once) have demonstrated the total accuracy of Marcelli's observations (above all in the fields of dermatology and allergology). I was able to verify (using two different bioelectronic tests, one from vibrational medicine and the other a bioelectrical impedance analysis) the local variation in electrical energy in the active points, with energy surges in the case of 'negative' points and falls in relation to positive points. It is very also helpful in the field of auricular diagnostics and therapy. I used the Test on various occasions on points outside the channels (rhinofacial puncture points, hand points and foot points) and I noticed how they corresponded to indications reported in both Chinese and European treatises.

Ultimately, the argument is so logically consistent and so well articulated that one could have an inkling (reasonable suspicion) of fraud. The internal secretion point (apex of the anti-tragus) is very important in existing conditions of chronic dermatosis (eczema, atopic dermatitis, psoriasis, vitiligo), as are the gall bladder point (on the top edge of the actual nose bone) in relation to ongoing urticaria and relapsing herpes, the lung point (on the bridge of the nose) for recent dermopathy and the kidney point (tip of the nose) for chronic dermopathy.

I have also verified the presence of the active points (positive and negative) on the auricular points (identified by Nogier and Bourdiol) of the upper limbs (scaphoid recess) and lower limbs (fossa navicularis) for ongoing chronic nummular eczema localised, as said, on the upper and lower limbs. Among the canonic points (not mentioned by Marcelli) I have often noticed the positivity of SI-7 Zhizheng (5 cun above the wrist, along a line connecting Yanggu with Xiaohai) in cases of chronic dermopathy linked to anxiety or relational disorders, and also of various Jueyin points (especially LR-3, LR-6 and PC-6) for ongoing 'lichen ruber planus' (three observations). Furthermore, I have been able to confirm (thanks to the Test) the hypothesis that the yuan and luo points are particularly indicated for mental disorders: the former for senility and/or disorders caused by reaction to the environment, the latter for predominantly juvenile endogenous situations.

In conclusion, after resigning myself to the idea of constantly having to pursue the truth without ever reaching it (the scepsis of doubt that Seneca talked about), Marcelli's book has brought me over to the side of 'positive doubt', of the Zeteticism of Bryson of Heraclea and of the *epoché*, which consists in a 'healthy suspension of judgement'. Books like this one allow us to discriminate between truth and untruth, between research and magic, between science and shamanism. In truth, magic and medicine were closely related or even identified with each other in the past, so much so that the mystery which surrounds life and its rules has been linked to all those traditional and passionate practices that were the foundations of magic and alchemy.

But in his book, Marcelli reminds us how a scientist must behave even when dealing with 'energy': before dividing up the various scientific fields, he should deal syncretically with physics, chemistry, philosophy and thus conduct a broad-ranging analysis of the multi-faceted, indefinable essence of biological phenomena.

The ultimate goal (and I can confirm that it is wholly reached) is not so much to find 'the philosopher's stone of sacred oriental medicine', but rather to elaborate a theory (by practical deduction) born of direct observation and experimentation, a formula which explains (in a wise and balanced way) the (dis)function of 'energy points'.

If it is true (as medical historians have noted) that from 1500 onwards science has moved ever farther away from magic to become its 'antithesis', it is moreover true that medical people remain firmly linked to 'magical-esoteric' subjects, which toss and turn in them like 'ghosts from an arcane and unconquerable past'. Marcelli's book gives us peace, puts our ghosts to rest and makes us understand a phenomenal truth which is at once humanist and scientific, a truth which supports (no less than other important western studies by Potigny, Pomeranz, Cantoni, Dumitrescu, Ionescu-Tergoviste, Bossy, etc) that which the Chinese classics had intuitively understood 30 centuries ago. To paraphrase Claudine Brelet-Rueff (an anthropologist from WHO and an expert in 'traditional medicine'), if it is true that the sacred medical arts contain the most ancient knowledge, the fruits of a search for harmony between inner life and external reality, this centuries-old experience must now be analysed in the light of more modern knowledge. Only in this way can that which might seem anecdotal, curious or the stuff of legend be classified (or re-classified) as scientific.

I wish the best of luck to this illuminating, courageous book, invaluable for its transparent simplicity, and like Tertullian I conclude: 'Habent sua fata libelli – Books have their destiny.'

Carlo Di Stanislao – L'Aquila, 31 August 1994

Umberto Mazzanti

A traditionally trained acupuncturist, physiatrist and sports medicine practitioner, Vice President of the Associazione Medici Agopuntori Bolognesi, formerly Vice President of the Società Italiana di Agopuntura, teacher and head of the Italo-Chinese school of acupuncture in Bologna.

The diagnostic-therapeutic method devised by Dr Marcelli and called the Active Points Test is characteristic of all empirical discoveries: it is simple, easy to use and effective.

On the one hand, it solves many of the problems of differential diagnosis when identifying a symptom's main aetiology, allowing us to verify the most important acupoint for solving the problem. On the other hand, it also provides us with the best point combinations so as not disturb the energy balance established by the initial penetration of the needle. Indeed, points that are found to be 'positive' during the first examination do not always remain so if they are put in combination with each other; in fact, they can become 'neutral' and even 'negative'. In my experience, these are the two fundamental aspects of the Test.

The Active Points Test demonstrates another important fact: it recognises in the skin, even when touched lightly, the ability to distinguish and evaluate, like a group of peripheral terminals connected to a central computer, not only the kind of sensation experienced, but also its hidden information, that is to say the true deeper message, and to decide on the most appropriate course for resolving the body's disorder.

This confirms our conviction, moreover shared by all those who practise acupuncture, that our bodies are always conscious of their own health status and often possess the instruments needed to combat the conditions that afflict them. Our job is to input, using a needle, the initial information that will activate their own capabilities.

With respect and gratitude.

Umberto Mazzanti – Bologna, 4 November 1994

Carlo Maria Giovanardi

A traditionally trained acupuncturist, President of the Associazione Medici Agopuntori Bolognesi and of the Fondazione Matteo Ricci, a teacher at the Italo-Chinese school of acupuncture, he has made numerous contributions to acupuncture research, including those of a modern scientific nature.

The thing that struck me most about Dr Marcelli's method is the collaborative relationship that is created between doctor and patient. Asking the patient if the symptom changes during the search for 'positive' points makes him/her a part of the process and contributes to the effectiveness of acupuncture.

The information which the practitioner gains from the Test is just as important.

Establishing a strategy for choosing the points to be used is fundamental to the success of therapy. I have personally noticed that, after selecting points on the basis of an energy diagnosis according to the rules of Traditional Chinese Medicine, this Test allows the practitioner to reduce even further the number of points, thus choosing only the most effective and discarding those that would 'disturb' the therapeutic effect. By this I mean that the Test takes on a clarifying role in many cases where it is extremely difficult to propose a definite diagnosis. The concurrence of points which are found to be effective by using both the Active Points Test and a traditional diagnostic process is also suggestive. This is confirmation that, rather than one model being more valid than another, what is often more important is the strictness with which it is applied.

Dr Carlo Maria Giovanardi – Bologna, 4 November 1994

Francesco Ceccherelli

A researcher at the Istituto di Anestesiologia e Rianimazione dell'Università di Padova, an acupuncturist and neuroreflexologist, Vice President of the Associazione Italiana per la Ricerca e l'Aggiornamento Scientifico (AIRAS), and author of numerous works of great scientific value.

Dear Marcelli,

Please allow me to give you my first impressions concerning the use of the so-called 'Active Points Test' that you recently proposed to me.

I want to make it clear first that, at this moment in time, I am not able to give you a proper structured account of my experiences showing false positive and negative results. Obviously, while using surface stimulation to search for distal points which modulate the patient's symptomatology, I have not explored all the points contained in the table you sent to me.

In view of the experimental model I chose, almost obligatorily given the nature of the Test, I systematically explored some of the so-called command points, some extra points and the contralateral homometameric segmental points. The patients examined using this method were suffering from pain due to deafferentation caused by nerve damage, postherpetic neuralgia or traumatic amputation. These are all forms of damage which cause severe, chronic pain that is always present. I was able to verify the differences in the patients' clinical history relative to the location of one or more the active points.

It appears that there are some points (the so-called active points) that produce a fleeting, momentary but real improvement in the medical condition, even when they are only stimulated at the surface, while stimulation of the majority of points does not produce any variation at all in the symptomatology.

As for the Test's mode of action, I do not believe it is necessary to rack one's brains to find an imaginative explanation; puncturing even the surface of the skin is certainly capable of activating the mechanonociceptors which are at the heart of the acupuncture effect when needles are inserted and stimulated in the usual way. Light and momentary stimulation of this kind, although it may not seem to be therapeutic in itself, is capable of generating interference at the posterior horn at a level somewhere between algogenic afferents and acupuncture afferents. If the point is 'active', or rather therapeutically useful, the patient will notice a slight variation in the symptom and this will allow the doctor to understand or rather foresee that stronger stimulation of the same point may have a role to play in therapy.

We must not forget that it has been proved for years that the therapeutic effect of acupuncture is principally due to the stimulation of the nociceptive mechanoreceptors whose central afferent is connected via the Aδ fibres. These nociceptors have a high threshold and adapt slowly or not at all; this means that the receptor discharges when energy that is potentially damaging to the body is applied, and stops discharging only when the tissue has been destroyed.

In the case of the Active Points Test, external stimulation with the tip of a needle, which the patient perceives as a light puncture and a slight pain, is in fact nociceptive stimulation of such receptors. It is, therefore, perfectly understandable for the symptom to show a subjective variation in intensity, albeit brief and fleeting. From my limited experience of this test and with carefully selected patients, it seems to me that it is particularly effective for identifying the 'active' segmental points. In my opinion, it is a little less certain when distal points are to be identified. However, I have already stated that I have limited experience with patients who are particularly demanding from a clinical point of view. This test is certainly innovative in terms of a clinical procedure for determining a set of acupoints to puncture during therapy.

Assuming that it proves its validity in a more robust and definitive experiment, the Test could represent an alternative to classical, traditional theory, which is based on an obsolete, theoretical and non scientific corpus, or even the consolidation of the reflex therapy model of acupuncture which since its birth has been based on the individualisation of a point's 'activity' through manual manipulation: pinching a fold of skin, exerting pressure or through its reaction to pain etc. The only intrinsic limit to the Active Points Test lies in the need for the patient's symptomatology to be present at the moment when the Test is carried out, as otherwise it is not possible to do it. This restricts its use to the more acute conditions or to those which are chronic but experiencing a flare-up at the time in question. It remains an interesting working hypothesis that all fellow acupuncturists should examine, verify and subsequently use in their clinical practice.

Dr Francesco Ceccherelli – Padua, 30 January 1995

Luciano Bassani

A physiatrist, neuro-reflexologist and colleague of Bourdio. In Italy he is an authority on vertebral manipulation, the author of some noteworthy articles and books and a teacher at the Centro Studi Terapie Naturali e Fisiche in Turin.

In his work *The Active Points Test*, Dr Marcelli has developed a diagnostic methodology which is of great interest and easy to learn.

Confronted with a patient, once the practitioner has gone through the traditional diagnostic procedure, he or she must move on to a programme of therapy; if neuro-reflex treatment is chosen, the choice must be directed towards what is suitable for the patient in question, as there is no doubt that therapy cannot be (and must never be) standardised, since not all patients will find treatment of the same areas and points effective.

Generally speaking, a comprehensive diagnostic approach should be used, taking into account all useful methods of investigation, in order to arrive at the right therapy plan. It is therefore necessary to subject the patient to an anthropometric examination to evaluate his constitution and to examine his iris in order to determine diathesis from its texture and sympathetic or parasympathetic dominance from the angle of Fuchs. Once these and any other diagnostic tests that are considered necessary have been carried out, and if neuro-reflex therapy is decided on, the next problem will be to choose the most appropriate neuro-reflex points.

It is for this particular reason that I consider my colleague Marcelli's Active Points Test to be a quick and helpful method that does not require the use of sophisticated equipment. When indicated, this test will finally help the practitioner to avoid savagely inserting needles in a search for those few points that are useful and sufficient for treatment. And this is very important as it is a further step towards attributing to acupuncture, and to other reflex therapies in general, the scientific value they deserve.

I would like to say a sincere thank you to Dr Marcelli.

Dr Luciano Bassani – Milan, 14 February 1995

Secondo Scarsella

An odontostomatologist and maxillofacial surgeon, traditional acupuncturist and reflexologist. He organises courses in TCM held by recognised and reputable teachers, and is the Science Director of the professional journal YI DAO ZHA ZI.

Dear Marcelli,

I am happy to inform you about the success of the Test which you devised.

I can imagine how, like all innovations, it must have met with scepticism from some quarters and with approval from others: please consider me among the latter.

Those of us who come from the Chinese school of acupuncture, like yours truly, are well aware that a lucky touch for acupoints is fundamental for obtaining optimal therapeutic results, but the same argument is considered to be of main importance in reflexology as well. I am therefore convinced that this 'intuition' of yours will be of great help to those of our colleagues who are new to the field and, as such, have understandable doubts; consequently it would not be a bad idea to introduce it into the syllabus of acupuncture courses. As far as my own specific field is concerned, I can report that I have experimented with your test in relation to acute dental conditions and facial algia and have found it to be reliable.

I wish you all the best while I await further developments.

Dr Secondo Scarsella – L'Aquila, 21 February 1995

Adolfo Panella

A specialist in Hygiene and Preventive Medicine, an acupuncturist trained in reflexology and a member of the Società Italiana di Riflessoterapia, Agopuntura Auricoloterapia (SIRAA).

Dear Stefano,

In my opinion, the Active Points Test has the potential to be a very useful method for investigating the correct course of therapy for conditions which are both kinesiologic and otherwise. It seems to me that two points should be underlined: the importance of the patient's clear perception of the symptom and the necessity of restricting to a minimum the number of points to be tested. On average, I believe that the limit should be 4–5 points at any one time. My impression is that if this limit is exceeded, even though he may still be collaborating, the patient will no longer be able to provide any useful answers. I believe that this is our cue for experimenting with and improving the Test's methodology.

I congratulate you and await future updates.

Best regards,

Adolfo Panella – Salerno, 22 February 1995

Julian N. Kenyon

A lecturer in anatomy and embryology at the University of Liverpool and founder of the British Medical Acupuncture Association, author of meticulous research intended to demonstrate the correctness of TCM and of the book 'Modern Techniques of Acupuncture', which has been translated into many languages.

I read Stefano Marcelli's work about the Active Points Test with interest. It is clearly a very practical and sensitive test which may be of enormous benefit, as long as the patient has symptoms which can be communicated while it is being performed. It may be widely used for these kinds of disorders. It could be carried out more effectively if taught directly, and for this reason I am happy to learn that Dr Marcelli organises training courses on it.

Dr Julian Kenyon – Southampton, 27 February 1995

Alberto Lomuscio
A cardiologist and traditional acupuncturist, Secretary of the Società Italiana di Agopuntura (SIA) and President of the Associazione Lombarda Medici Agopuntori (ALMA).

Dear Dr Marcelli,

I was very pleased to receive your interesting book about the Active Points Test, which I read with great care. With regard to this original method of non-invasive acupuncture diagnosis, I am happy to report the following:

1. The Test shows a solid connection with Traditional Chinese Acupuncture, whose most traditional rational principles it never distorts, and has been conceived in line with the main classical texts of TCM

2. The fact that it is extremely easy to use makes it accessible to any practitioner capable of practising acupuncture, without adding at all to the average time required for a sitting but notably enriching those diagnostic abilities which derive from the traditional methods currently in use (energy case history, tongue or pulse examination etc.)

3. I have personally tested the effectiveness of the Test on dozens of patients, affected by a wide variety of energy conditions, and I have noticed a high level of correspondance between the results of this Test and a diagnosis obtained using traditional methods: in the cases that I studied this correspondance was close to 100%. Furthermore, I noted that the more positive the point's reaction was to the Test, the more effective this point proved to be in subsequent needle therapy

4. Given the Test's excellent sensitivity, I would like to propose a further improvement to the Test itself, that is the future possibility of 'grading' its diagnostic sensibility with the aim of creating a priority treatment scale for acupoints should many of them react positively to the Test at the same time.

Best regards,

Dr Alberto Lomuscio – Milan, 15 March 1995

Natour Mohammad
A specialist in general haematology and an expert in acupuncture, homeopathy and iridology. He is the Founder and President of the Associazione Medici Agopuntori Liguri (AMAL).

I learned of the Active Points Test technique in December 1994 and I immediately started to use it, selecting the most complicated cases I had in my surgery up to 15 March 1995. I employed the method in 250 cases, divided as follows:

- 100 cases of cervical syndrome and/or stiffness of the neck
- 50 cases of lumbosciatalgia and/or disc herniation
- 30 cases of coxalgia from arthrosis and/or osteoporosis
- 30 cases of headache and/or migraine
- 12 cases of allergic rhinitis and/or allergic asthma
- 10 cases of tachycardia (anxiety-depression syndrome)
- 10 cases of neuralgia (trigeminal, Zoster and intercostal)
- 5 cases of gastralgia
- 3 cases of nausea and vomiting.

Based on my personal experience, I can confirm the validity of the method of choosing so-called ++ points.

When carrying out the Test, I have come across very few negative points and a considerable number of neutral points (which, unfortunately, I did not count). I have employed this method with great enthusiasm as it has given me the chance to involve the patient him/herself, not only by making the patient concentrate on the symptom which affects him/her, but also by getting him/her to notice in a tangible and subjective way how valid and effective the acupuncture therapy with which he/she is being treated really is.

In conclusion, I invite all my colleagues who are experts in energy medicine (especially Traditional Chinese Medicine) to explore this methodology in order to develop it, as I am sure that we are only at the inception of a safe method for confirming the diagnosis of the Traditional Chinese Medicine 'specialist'.

Dr Mohammad Natour – Genoa, 17 March 1995

Stefano Crispini

A traditional acupuncturist, student of Professor Nguyen Tai Thu, and Scientific Director of the Associazione Medici Agopuntori Liguri (AMAL).

After using it numerous times I have concluded that, if performed correctly, the Test proposed by Dr Marcelli will always give true results.

It will help those who are a little too eager and assume that twenty acupoints might be useful when they can use only five, and it will help the less able or decisive, who really do not know which path to follow. In any case, the Test will provide reliable support to all practitioners in terms of both diagnosis and therapy.

Its true value lies in its simplicity.

Dr Stefano Crispini – Genoa, 21 March 1995

Gérard Guillaume

A rheumatologist, traditional acupuncturist and reflexologist, teacher at various schools and author of some important research, numerous articles and books about acupuncture, and a prominent member of the Association Française d'Acupuncture (AFA).

Dear Dr Marcelli,

I have just finished reading your manuscript. I am sorry I was not able to do it earlier but, due to my many commitments, I have very little time available. I want to congratulate you on your work, which bridges the gap between acupuncture and reflexology and which brings with it interesting opportunities. It demonstrates, if there were any need to do so, that research is still a topical issue in a thousand-year-old medical tradition. A more circumstantial opinion would require an experimental evaluation to be conducted systematically, which I believe to be possible. Please let me know if you wish to publish this work in France.

Best regards,

Dr Gérard Guillaume – Paris, 26 March 1995

Jean-Pierre Multedo

A French mesotherapist, author of books translated into Italian and Spanish, 'maître de stage' of the Societé Française de Mésothérapie, and President of the Groupe Méditérraneen de Mésothérapie.

My colleague Dr Stefano Marcelli, as a sign of friendship, has done me the honour of asking my opinion as a mesotherapist on his Active Points Test. As I have no specific qualification in Acupuncture, it is difficult for me to appreciate fully the Test's value in this field. Nevertheless, reading his work has allowed me to further my understanding of the neurophysiological processes of the various reflex therapies. Dr Marcelli possesses such an ability to summarize and writes with such clarity that I was immediately tempted to try out his Test in mesotherapy.

As its inventor, Dr Michel Pistor, said, mesotherapy is a *'new therapeutic idea that allows us to move the location of therapy nearer to the location of the disease'*. It is a localised pharmacological form of therapy, performed on a vertical line from the diseased area, intradermically or in the upper layer of the subcutis.

But, through practice, we have found that mesotherapy is also a very important means of treating certain medical conditions that are further away from the site of the injection. For this reason it would fall within the definition of reflex therapy: *'A method that consists in the distal treatment of disease, using the skin as a switch and inducing stimulation or anaesthesia at the cutaneous projection regions of the organs affected.'*

So, like Dr Marcelli, we believe that it is possible to include mesotherapy among the reflex therapies and to apply to it the general principles that govern those practices, that is to say the search for and treatment of so-called 'active' points.

In mesotherapy we have listed a certain number of specific points and areas for each condition. They are:

- first of all, those indicated spontaneously by the patient

- next, those which we locate using palpation or the *palper rouler*

- then, those that are stimulated by active or passive counter-resistance manoeuvres

- lastly, points which can be distal indications of disease, and whose topography is borrowed from other therapies (Valleix points, acupuncture points, auricular points, etc.).

There is no reason not to treat these points when the situation merits it, and it seems to us that the Active Points Test is an originally helpful method for testing them and will constitute an important step forward in our daily practice.

For my part, I have begun to use it successfully in relation to certain common conditions, such as sciatic or cervicobrachial neuralgia. It allows us to know if we should treat or not treat, if we should inject without hesitation or not inject a product that could be uselessly painful; hence the advantages are that it is effective and saves time. I therefore believe that Dr Marcelli's method should be incorporated into our therapeutic practices *in so far as we consider mesotherapy to constitute not just a simple form of local therapy but also a form of 'wet reflex therapy'*.

Dr Jean-Pierre Multedo – Le Cannet, 26 March 1995

Vito Marino

A traditional acupuncturist, President of the Associazione Culturale 'Qi' and Head of the Scuola di Medicina Tradizionale Cinese in Palermo.

Dear Stefano,

I have recently had the opportunity to try your Active Points Test and, despite the exiguity of my case study, my impression is that of a fairly reliable technique capable of 'predicting' the effectiveness of selected points.

In two cases in particular, one of back pain caused by paravertebral contracture and one of migraine crisis, the Test was so effective that I was able to select a group of acupoints which brought about the nullification of the symptomology as soon as the needles had been applied.

Best regards,

Vito Marino – Palermo, 5 October 1995

Franco Cracolici

A traditional acupuncturist and Head of the Scuola di Agopuntura Tradizionale in Florence.

Dear Marcelli,

I must tell you that I have tried the Active Points Test and I have found your book to be intuitive and to provide the kind of classification that many acupuncturists probably had at heart but were not able to formulate.

In my opinion the following points are very important: the difference in the way the symptom is perceived, the testing of distal points and the doctor–patient relationship, in which the skin acts as intermediary between the two energy levels (Doctor and Patient).

The Active Points Test's greatest contribution to Medicine is, in fact, that it does not rush in blindly. It represents the rediscovery of the Art of Medicine, based on the location of the active points (whether they are negative, positive or indifferent), which should be operated on with patience. In my opinion, an example of this is the opening of the Key Points on the Curious Channels and of the Window of the Sky Points, which require particular attention.

I have also noticed that sometimes the *palper rouler* may be useful as a precursor to the needle test. In any case, as is written in the ancient texts: *'In order to puncture a point well, you first need to knock and if this is done gently, the door will open.'*

So, Marcelli, I thank you for your contribution to Traditional Chinese Medicine.

Franco Cracolici – Florence, 12 October 1995

And, *dulcis in fundo*:

Alessandra Gulì

A traditional acupuncturist and herbalist and a teacher at numerous schools throughout Italy and abroad. She is a prominent member of various acupuncture and Chinese phytotherapy associations, as well as an honorary professor at the College of Traditional Chinese Medicine at the University of Nanjing.

Dear Stefano,

I am sending you, as promised, some notes on my brief experience with your acupuncture examination method. My response has not been delayed by disinterest but rather by my busy lifestyle. I try to follow the harmony of Chinese philosophy and do fewer things than I would like, so as to protect the quality of my work and to reduce stress to a minimum, because, if *we* live frenetic lives, how can we be convincing when we encourage patients to regulate *their* lives? I will now describe some of the impressions I gained from using the Test you introduced me to and which you have asked my opinion about, and I want to thank you for your faith in me.

I was able to use the Active Points Test in nine cases, but without verifying it over time or making a comparative analysis with similar cases in which it was not used. These few cases were, nevertheless, all quite significant. It was possible to identify 'positive points' in all of them and 'negative points' in many. So, these points exist in my experience as well, and the reaction to their stimulation was quite evident. The symptomology of the patients concerned did not only include pain, but in some was quite different, for example: intense dizziness, feeling of emptiness in the stomach and gastrointestinal hypermotility not caused by hunger etc.

I found a great deal of agreement between the response of the points (positive, negative and indifferent) to the Test and the energy diagnosis, and at times stimulation of the points indicated by the Test can settle any doubts as to the diagnosis, whether related to the channels affected by the energy imbalance or to the sort of condition that is affecting them. The point's nature (positivity, negativity, indifference) could be a precise reflection of the condition of the body in accordance with the 'full–empty' contradiction, but I have not yet had an opportunity to go into this analysis in detail as regards the ambiguous cases. If this were really the case, then the population of Italy is in more of an 'empty state' than it appears to be, and much could be said and done about this.

When points which gave 'positive' results to the Test respond to actual puncture by significantly reducing symptoms during and at the end of the session, this is without doubt, as you yourself have suggested as regards the first sessions, an immediate and beneficial result. However, not having been able to follow up with these patients over time, I am not in a position to quantify the results with regard to the sessions during which the Test was not used (without the Test, the points varied by one or two units, but gave good results at the time and fair results with hindsight).

I have used 'positive' points with the reinforcing method and the uniform method (of harmonization), depending on the type of disharmony from the point of view of energy, but I have promised myself to use the reinforcing method in future (even in those cases where the uniform method might seem more appropriate to me). I have never used dispersion on a positive point, even in a case where I suspected it that it might be the best technique to adopt.

From the facts I have set out here, I can draw the following conclusions: when the surface of the skin is punctured, 'positive', 'negative' and 'indifferent' points really exist, and their puncturing provokes a precise reaction in the patients' symptomatology. The selection of these points rather than others during therapy constitutes an extremely interesting method which is worth experimenting more widely and in ways which are closely linked to the energy aspects of Traditional Chinese Medicine. In this sense it would be desirable to explore in more detail the relationship between the nature of the point (positive, negative or indifferent) and the needle manipulation technique.

So, 'Marcelli's Test' could be of great significance, not only as a guide to the choice of points, but also as a refinement of the diagnostic aspect of Traditional Chinese Medicine. For the moment, it will push us towards study and research, thus favouring an exchange of scientific ideas among those who are concerned with this medical 'discipline' and who practise it on a daily basis.

Best regards,

Dr Alessandra Gulì – Rome, 12 October 1995

THE ACTIVE POINTS TEST IN AURICULAR PUNCTURE

BY MARCO ROMOLI

PREFACE TO THE SECOND EDITION

I have drawn great satisfaction from my continued use of the Active Points Test over the years and I always offer it as part of my teaching courses. The Test is mentioned in chapter five of my book *Agopuntura auricolare*, UTET 2003 (pp. 60–63), as 'The Active Points or Needle Contact Test'. In my article about the use of the technique for identifying the most effective point for a migraine attack the Test is called the 'Needle Contact Test'. This is the title of chapter seven of the book *Auricular Acupuncture Diagnosis*, published by Churchill Livingstone (Elsevier) in 2009.

OUTLINE

I willingly agreed to examine some of my patients using my colleague Marcelli's test. From my very first observations I have considered it to be a very interesting method:

1. It is easy to execute even for acupuncturists who are just starting out.

2. It adapts very well to acupuncture of the ear because the whole body can be examined from a limited surface area like the auricle.

3. Using Marcelli's categorisation method (strongly positive, positive, indifferent and negative points) priority can be given during the examination to the most effective points for therapy.

In this way, the number selected will be limited to those which are indispensable (from one to a maximum of three according to my observations).

4. Patients who resort to acupuncture often present with an intricate symptomatology that dates back over time. In my opinion, Marcelli's method is excellent for 'breaking down' the clinical picture, implementing therapy in stages and for following up the patient's response to it over time. For example, I consider it to be very useful in the field of physiatry: at least one point resulting positive to the Test should correspond to each limited and painful movement (see Case 1 below).

5. Furthermore, as Marcelli has already mentioned, it appears that the Active Points Test will allow the identification of cases that are 'absolute non-responders' to acupuncture (rare) or that give a relative response (more frequent), when the Test works and there is a response to therapy but it is limited over time and does not show a progressive increase in wellbeing during successive sessions (see below in the discussion).

6. Last but not least, as Marcelli has pointed out, is the active participation in the diagnosis and therapy of the people we are examining. I have noticed that in general patients immediately grasp the significance of the Test and cooperate well. This participation is fundamental for their recovery and has a positive influence on the doctor–patient relationship.

Before talking about the method used in my case study, which was limited to 18 patients, I should mention *Auricular Therapy*, which is the term used by French authors, or more simply *Ear Acupuncture* as it has been called by the Chinese.

As we know, ear acupuncture is a recently developed method which is generally agreed to have been discovered by Dr Nogier (his first publications date from 1957) [1]. The method found fertile ground in China where in the 1970s and 1980s there was great interest and an eagerness to study it, which led progressively to an increase in the number of points studied [2, 3]. The ensuing 30 years of study and practice of the method have led to the consolidation of two schools, the French and the Chinese, which have both adopted auricle maps that partly overlap each other but that also vary in some aspects. There are no real contradictions, only different interpretations of the points [4]. While the western school insists there is a close relationship (possibly one to one) between the points and the structure of the anatomy, the Chinese, who in my opinion are more flexible, pay particular attention to the symptoms of bodily dysfunction which precede the appearance of the actual disease. There are those who argue that the Chinese could not help but be influenced by their traditional medicine. There is no doubt that, while western maps show one liver point, the Chinese ones have at least four, depending on whether the point relates to acute hepatitis, chronic hepatitis with hepatomegaly and/or cirrhosis, or to functions of the liver that regulate the production of marrow in the red corpuscles in cases of anaemia, muscle tone in musculoskeletal disorders or the health of the eyes.

Ear acupuncture has, in my opinion, great advantages:

1. simplicity of execution

2. speed and power of effect

3. as an emergency therapy it can be carried out in different locations and situations without the need for the patient to undress, saving time and space.

These advantages have often persuaded our colleagues to use the method together with somatic acupuncture. The method's difficulties are essentially as follows:

1. Positioning on the ear: the points and reflex areas are concentrated in a small space and there are not many anatomical trace reference points, unlike on the soma. That is why the Chinese have adopted simple maps using the names and depictions of anatomical parts.

2. Point size: points are smaller and distances of less than a millimetre can have an influence on the therapeutic effect. That is why points must be located carefully using the two methods available: electrical detection and pressure palpation.

3. The significance of finding a positive point with the two methods mentioned above. Initially, we will only be able to make a 'topographic' diagnosis; for example if the stomach point is found to be sensitive, we will know that this area has

a problem whose ethiopathogenesis we are unaware of, but we will know that we must evaluate it using every means at our disposal (medical case history, laboratory tests, X-rays of the digestive system, endoscopy, etc.). On the other hand, referring to the stomach point on the map as the direct projection of the viscera on the auricle may lead to error. In the opinion of some authors such as Jarricot, the auricular points are the projection of the nervous system of that organ or of the plexus or ganglion that innervates parts it [5, 6]. The above-mentioned author has proposed an interesting diagnostic method which consists in making reflex dermatalgia disappear by stimulating the tip of the auricle through massage or the use of electrical current of low intensity;

4. Last but by no means less important for diagnosis and therapy is the notion of laterality. In somatic acupuncture it is not often taken into consideration because, save for a few exceptions, channels are usually punctured bilaterally. On the auricle, however, curious phenomena of unilateral point distribution are often observed and do not only appear in the stress response [7]. For example, in cases of cervicalgia, headache or pharyngitis which present with clear bilateral pain distribution, we may find sensitive points on one auricle only. Treatment of that side alone will be enough to reduce bilateral pain.

EXAMINATION OF THE AURICLE AND APPLICATION OF THE TEST

Dr Marcelli examined the ear using the most well-known method, that is to say locating points that are sensitive to pressure with a probe, an empty ballpoint pen or a spring-loaded *palpeur* calibrated to a constant pressure of between 150 g and 400 g, depending on which instrument is used.

This is a valid method in which the point to be punctured can be located with precision. Once the point has been found, the Test is performed and positive or strongly positive points are selected for therapy (see below for action regarding negative points). I have always considered the search for a sensitive point and its subsequent massage to be of great diagnostic importance: in order to correlate clearly a symptom to an auricular point, it must be possible to alter the intensity and topography of somatic or visceral pain, the contraction of a muscle group or the sensitivity of reflex dermatalgia by massaging the point for 30–60 seconds with an instrument.

This type of massage is always quite painful. I have noticed that the Active Points Test is quicker (by two to three seconds) and does not generally cause pain. The tip of a needle is more effective, therefore, than the rounded end of a palpation instrument.

The other method of studying the auricle is through electrical detection. As all acupuncturists know, this consists in exploring the cutis with low intensity electrical current in the search for points which are less resistant to electricity than the skin which surrounds them; these generally correspond to the points which are classically situated on the acupuncture channels.

The ear behaves in a similar way and there are always a few positive points that can be detected even in apparently healthy subjects. These combinations vary and will depend on the ongoing symptomatology and medical history of the patient being examined. Electrical detection is not an absolutely conclusive method and is affected by a few factors that are not unimportant, such as dampness of the skin, emotional tension in the patient etc. Despite these limitations, it remains an irreplaceable method for the work of acupuncturists. In research that I have been pursuing for some time, I have been using a combination of both methods to examine my patients, starting with electrical detection and following this up with palpation. This gives me the following possibilities for each point:

1. the point gives a positive result to electrical detection and a negative one to palpation;

2. the point gives a positive result to both electrical detection and palpation;

3. the point gives a negative result to electrical detection but is sensitive to palpation.

Groups 1) and 2) occur with the same frequency but in my opinion have different meanings; while the points in group 1) refer to prior medical conditions and/or symptoms of secondary importance, the points in group 2) are characteristic of an ongoing condition and are useful for therapy (and also frequently give positive results to the Active Points Test). Group 3), which is much less frequent, generally appears at the end of a session during which part of the symptomatology still persists. So careful palpation of the entire area of the auricle relating to pain symptoms must be repeated. If necessary, the sensitivity of auricular points corresponding to the internal organs that may cause related pain in that area or on the acupuncture channels that cross it should be checked. In this way, a final point which is very sensitive to palpation and often gives strongly positive results to this Test can be highlighted. So with regard to gonalgia with no real clinical indications that the joint is involved and with very few or no indications from radiology, the knee point (if positive) will be treated first. If the symptoms persist, even to a lesser degree, a careful check will be carried out of the sensitivity of the area of the lumbar rachis, the hip, the ovary, the spleen, the gall bladder etc. On this last sensitive point I often apply a permanent needle for a period of not less than 7–15 days.

In those cases where the Active Points Test was performed, presented below, I chose to use the electrical detection method only. Considering the delicate nature of Marcelli's Test, and the need for the patient's full cooperation, I wanted to eliminate all painful sensations during the course of the examination. Furthermore, given the complicated nature of the auricle's nervous system and its distinctive 'reflex genicity', I thought it would be a good idea to avoid using two different stimulation methods so that its sensitivity to the Active Points Test would not be changed excessively. One auricle must be completely explored with the detector before passing on to the other. Every positive point must be marked with a marker pen. The best way to explore the auricle is from the top to the bottom, for example in the following order: the antihelix, (superior and inferior root), the antihelix to the posterior auricular groove, the groove or recess of the helix from the top to the bottom, the helix from the top to the bottom towards the tail, the cymba conchae, the root and ascending branch of the helix, the cavum conchae with the intertragic notch, tragus, anti-tragus, the lateral and medial surface of the lobe and the entire medial surface of the auricle from the top to the bottom.

Particular attention should be given to the hidden areas, especially to the cymba and cavum conchae, the elective projection seats of the internal organs which often give positive results to electrical detection, as does the intertragic notch onto which important structures related to the hypothalamus and hypophysis are projected.

CASE STUDY

I examined 18 patients with this method: 8 males (with an average age of 41) and 10 females (with an average age of 44.9). The symptomatology presented was as follows:

- 2 patients with acute lumbalgia (back strain)

- 4 patients with chronic lumbalgia; 2 of these also suffered from headache, primarily related to tension in 1 case and due to miscellaneous causes in the other (Case 3)

- 2 patients with sciatica (Case 4)

- 2 patients with chronic tendonitis (thumb abductors, supraspinatus muscle in the shoulder)

- 1 patient with metatarsalgia

- 2 patients with cervicobrachialgia from discal uncoarthrosis and narrowing of the C5-C7 lower vertebral foramens (Case 1)

- 2 patients with neck pain and subjective vertigo as after-effects of cervical whip lash

- 1 patient with esophagitis (Case 2)

- 1 patient with acute sinusitis

- 1 patient suffering from the after-effects of an operation on popliteal cysts on the knee (troubling hyperesthesia of the popliteal hollow when lightly touched with a finger, excellent result with the Test).

The patients were examined during a minimum of three sittings a week for a total of 21 days. The results were as follows: a good response in 13 cases, with the same points also giving typically positive results to the Test in successive sittings. The response to therapy was good during the first week with the patient feeling better after four to six days and showing continued improvement during successive sittings. In one case of acute lumbalgia there was no response to the Test or to therapy (a young person of 23). The Test achieved no response from four different points, both before and after manipulation of the lower vertebral column. In four other patients the Test gave positive results but response to therapy did not last longer than a few hours (up to a maximum of 24–36 hours) after the first sitting and successive sittings did not prolong the period of wellbeing.

The positive nature of the points tested proved to be inconsistent during successive sittings (it was maintained in only two cases out of four). The medical case histories of this group, which I call the *relative non-responders*, were examined with a view to discovering any possible causes of interference such as septic foci in the dental arches or in any part of the cephalic area (paranasal sinuses, ears etc.), malocclusion, dysmetabolic states, food intolerance, the presence of 'active' scars etc.

In two cases, interference from the stomatognathic system was found (malocclusion in Case 4 and pericoronitis of the lower eighth, ipsilateral to cervicobrachialgia which was resistant to treatment with drugs. The Test achieved a positive response from the lower jaw point and the symptomatology responded well to the extraction of the tooth).

In two other cases which were similar to each other, lumbalgia and headache, intolerances to different foods were found (Case 3). A total of 70 points were examined with the Active Points Test. On a limited group of patients such as mine, I made the following observations:

1. An average of 3.9 points were tested for each patient, and at least 1.9 of those gave positive or strongly positive results. They typically remained positive when retested and the sequence of points was varied, they maintained their localisation in successive sittings and tended to become less positive as therapy took effect;

2. There were a slightly more limited number of indifferent points (1.5 per patient) and painful points (1.3 per patient). The latter appear with some frequency on the auricle and are useful for therapy. Looking for the most sensitive point has always been considered useful by Chinese authors and is achieved by lightly pricking one area of the auricle (see the reference to Soulie de Mourant on page 60) or by withdrawing the needle slightly and inserting it again at different angles. In my case study, the

painful points were counted but not subjected to the Test, so as not to interfere with the patient's perception of the pain caused by his symptoms;

3. There were certainly a more limited number of negative points (0.4 per patient) but in general they were clearly noticeable. Sometimes electrical detection may find two symmetrical points (although symmetry is not the rule in auricular puncture) which during the Test turn out to have the opposite polarity to the negative point which is ipsilateral or contralateral to the painful symptomatology, as in the case of lumbalgia in Case 3. I preferred not to puncture the negative points because the Chinese and French masters of auricular puncture do not describe reinforcing and dispersion techniques. It cannot be ruled out that these points might also be effective if we consider how responses to non-pharmacological therapies and to non-conventional methods of care can fluctuate. Doctors who are experts in this field know that these fluctuations are important and useful for achieving the patient's mental and physical wellbeing.

4. As for the points about which there is some doubt, when the patient says nothing or is slow to respond, more often than not it is because the points are indifferent.

   In my opinion, though, other ambiguous points can be found, especially after a ++ point: if the strongly positive point is found at the end of the examination, there will obviously be no problems with its evaluation, but if a point turns out to be ++ at the beginning or half way though the examination, in some cases the effect tends to continue for a while and to extend its positivity to the next few points (see Case 3).

   For this reason it is a good idea to wait for a few minutes, then locate the position or painful movement of the patient again and continue testing the remaining points. This delayed effect may be characteristic of the auricle and of its 'reflex genicity'. As a matter of fact, small stimuli from touch, heat and light etc are capable of varying the flow of sensory afferents towards the nerve structures of the encephalic trunk and the thalamocortex.

The four cases that follow are, in my opinion, the most interesting. Since we can all learn something from failure, I decided to recount the story of two of the Test's *relative non-responders* (Cases 3 and 4).

Case 1: C. Piero, age 67, businessman

No illnesses worthy of note. Suffered cervical whiplash two and a half years ago. At that time he had not been advised to wear a collar. After 7–8 months he started to suffer from recurring cervicobrachialgia with pain in the shoulder and in the left scapula. The symptoms were worsened by prolonged periods in the driving position, but responded well to NSAIDs.

He had been suffering from frequent neck pain with subjective vertigo without headaches for one year. The patient complained of constant soreness and contracture of the trapezius muscles and of the elevator muscle of the left scapula. Doppler US of the neck arteries within normal limits, standard and oblique projection X-rays of the cervical spine show discal uncoarthrosis of the lower cervical metamers with narrowing of the C5–C6, C6–C7 foramens, above all on the left side. I examined the cervical spine in movement: anteroflexion and lateroflexion on the left were noticeably limited and painful, less so on the right. Electrical detection found three points, on the left side only.

Numbers 1 and 2 are located immediately behind the helix and, according to Nogier, belong to the segmental distribution chain of the sympathetic spinal marrow nuclei (from C2 to Th11) [8], point number 3, on the other hand, in my opinion corresponds to the vertebral bodies of C6-C7 [4]. Point 2 was positive (+), but the point that stood out (++) was number 3: resting the needle on it and following the patient's movement led to freer anteroflexion and lateroflexion on the left (Figure A.1). Pain persisted in right lateroflexion after the needle was inserted. I rested the needle on point 2 and this movement became unobstructed as well.

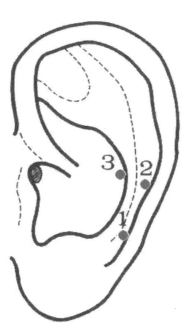

Figure A.1 Active Points Test on the ear to check the most effective points in a case of cervicobrachialgia with shoulder pain

Acupuncture on these two points gave the patient relief that lasted ten days. This combination was repeated in the two successive sittings with excellent results over time.

Case 2: B. Primo, age 57, bricklayer

Operations on a left and right inguinal hernia 25 years before. He had been suffering from sero-negative rheumatoid arthritis for 20 years. At various times he had been treated with gold salt therapy, metothrexate and recently with cortisone and NSAIDs. Gastroduodenitis for three to four years (X-ray diagnosis); three to four month history of epigastralgia and retrosternal burning with little response to gastroprotective therapy with antacids and anti-receptors. The patient had already completed a few courses of auricular puncture with good results in relation to the painful symptoms, oedema in the hands and mobility of the metacarpal-phalangeal joints. I examined the patient's auricles with the electrical detector and found points on the cymba and cavum conchae (four on the right and three on the left) which I subjected to the Test (Figure A.2). However, when he was examined, the patient was asymptomatic; I then asked him to locate a painful point in the area where his symptoms usually manifested. The patient located one which responded painfully to pressure on the midline corresponding to the xiphoid process. I explained the Active Points Test to him; while I examined his auricles with the tip of a needle, he should indicate to me whether there was any variation in the pain response to pressure. I expected point number 1, the bilateral point relating to the duodenum, to be positive but, contrary to my expectations, it was indifferent. Points 2 and 3 on the right (the esophagus and the adrenal gland according to the Chinese) and 2 and 3 on the left (stomach and Triple Heater to the Chinese) were also indifferent. Only point 3 on the right gave a clear response (++).

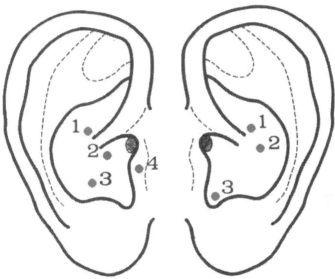

Figure A.2 Active Points Test on the ear
Points that practitioners expect to be active can result inactive and vice versa.

I waited for a few minutes and then I re-tested the points in a different sequence: point 3 was still the only positive point. On the maps there is no mention of points that are connected to the digestive system in that area of the auricle, but Jarricot [5, 9] links it to dermatalgia of the fifth dorsal dermatome which includes point 1, the area relating to anxiety. In my experience [10], point 3 should relate to gastroesophageal reflux and/or incontinence of the LES with distal esophagitis. As often happens when different maps of the ear are consulted as in this case, there do not appear to be real differences of opinion but simply different interpretations. Inserting the needle into this point completely eliminated the painful reaction to pressure on the xiphoid process. Extracting the needle produced a moderate amount of bleeding, which to the Chinese is an important sign that the therapy is effective. The improvement in the patient's condition lasted all week and at the second sitting I discovered that point 3 on the right and point 2 on the left (stomach) were still positive. After 20 days the symptoms were in remission but another few sessions were still required.

Case 3: M. Gabriella, age 50, office worker

This patient's medical history is full and includes: familial hypercholesterolemia and diabetes, operation on an umbilical hernia and appendicitis at age 7, tonsillectomy at age 9, cholecystectomy at age 29 for cholesterol stones. In addition, she had had three miscarriages when she was 31, an ovariotomy and left tube resection due to an ill-defined adnexitis and tubo-ovarian abscess, an operation on an anal fistula at age 38, and phlebitis in the right leg at age 40 with residual venous insufficiency. She was allergic to nickel and to some medications such as aspirin and Novalgin. She had been suffering from migraines for 20 years; at first they had been very intense and frequent (every two to three days) accompanied by vomiting and photophobia. However, during the last ten years they had improved and at the time were occurring, without vomiting, only once or twice a month, above all during menstruation. Pain from the migraines had always been located in the temporal region, in the parietal, mastoid and nuchal regions.

The patient had tried acupuncture twice and had found it beneficial. However, for a few months she had been suffering from a different headache which she described as a continuous feeling of heaviness on both sides of the vertex and the forehead, which forced her to close her eyes often and made it difficult to concentrate. The physiological medical history showed that the patient had complained of colitis and episodes of diarrhoea, dyspepsia with a bitter taste in the mouth and post-prandial abdominal distension. It was interesting to note that, in the morning on an empty stomach, she felt fine and her problems began only when she started to eat something. Initially the patient was requesting acupuncture treatment for gonalgia, the after-effect of a distortion injury which had occurred one year before, and for rachiodynia at the level of the cervix and above all at the lumbar spine with lower back pain and sciatica on the left side, all of which had been troubling her for at least 10 years.

An X-ray of the lumbar spine showed a slight scoliotic deviation with discopathy at L4–L5. I examined the whole of her vertebral column and in particular the lumbosacral spine: osteo-tendon reflexes present and symmetrical, Lasègue sign was negative, sensitivity was normal. The patient did not complain of sciatica but of lower back pain which occurred during stretching movements while standing. Using the electrical detector, I found two symmetrical points on the lower branch of the antihelix corresponding to the projection of the gluteal muscles (according to the Chinese) or of the sacroiliac joint (according to the French).

Resting the needle on the point on the left side, I followed the patient's lumbar spine extension movement. The pain worsened and the patient's sciatica returned. I repeated the manoeuvre on the contralateral side, which was usually asymptomatic, and the pain disappeared (++). I punctured the right side only and the effect was maintained for the whole of the session; at the end of it I performed lumbar spine flexion manipulation in accordance with Maigne's no-pain rule. The patient was well for the whole week and I repeated the same manoeuvre during the second session, stabilising the effect.

At the third sitting, the patient was complaining of a headache and a sensation of heavy-headedness extending from the crown to the forehead and eyes. Using the detector, I found six points on the left and four on the right (Figure A.3). The Test gave the following results in this order: on the left, point 1 was negative, 2 was indifferent, 3 was indifferent, 4 was indifferent, 5 was +, 6 was indifferent; on the right, point 1 was painful, 2 and 3 were ++, 4 was impossible to evaluate (ambiguous).

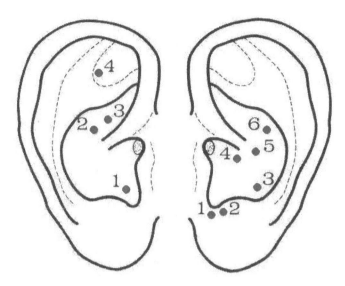

Figure A.3 Active Points Test on the ear in a case of chronic back pain due to discopathy at L4-L5

During the testing of points 2 and 3 on the right (Liver and Gall Bladder according to Jarricot) the patient's headache eased considerably and inserting the needles prolonged this effect. The patient began to feel drowsy and the headache moved to the left temple (the usual site of her migraine). I repeated the Test on point 5 of the left auricle (Stomach according to the Chinese, celiac plexus for Jarricot) which now gave me a ++ response and the pain in her temple disappeared. The effect of this therapy was strong and was maintained for about 2 days. It is interesting to note that points 1 and 2 on the left (eye and forehead area for the Chinese), which are generally useful for the treatment of migraines, were not so for this particular headache. On the contrary, point 1 actually made it worse.

The patient returned for the next session with the same headache. The Test achieved the same response from the usual points. This was repeated at the third session. The therapy worked but its effect did not last for the whole period between one session and another, which is one of the basic parameters for evaluating the effectiveness of acupuncture treatment. Given that the three effective points all belonged to the digestive area and taking into account the chronic nature of the dyspepsia and irritable colon, I suggested to the patient that it would be a good idea to conduct some research on food intolerance using a variation of the method of Gianfranceschi and colleagues [11].

Tests showed a marked intolerance to beef, milk and dairy products, less for eggs, wheat and maize. I suggested to the lady that she give up these foods for 2–3 months. After 20 days, the patient's digestive problems and headache showed a marked improvement and menstruation with regular blood flow had occurred without being accompanied by migraine, which had not happened for a long time. In this case, the Test was useful principally as an instrument of differential diagnosis.

Case 4: P. Monia, age 25, secretary

She worked for long hours at the computer with her head rotated to the right. Hepatitis A at age eight. No other serious illnesses or symptoms worthy of note. At age 20 she suffered an injury to her right knee following a fall from a scooter. There were no apparent lasting consequences. For two to three years the patient had been complaining of almost continual bilateral rigidity of the cervix with hypersensitivity to cold and draughts. Cervicalgia was accompanied by a tension-type headache with aching and tension in the masseteric, periauricular and bilateral temporal region. These disorders were worse in the evening after a day's work and were periodically accompanied by a feeling of disorientation. The patient slept regularly and did not seem particularly anxious. She sometimes had a tendency to clench her teeth. Her first episode of right-sided sciatica was four months earlier. She had been well over the summer. At the end of September, the sciatica had returned together with lower back pain which would manifest just before daybreak. She slept on an orthopaedic mattress and used a high pillow. At the consultation she presented with negative Lasègue sign, osteo-tendon reflexes of the lower limbs were present and symmetrical, there were no sensitivity disorders. The lumbar spine was painful when extended and during left lateroflexion, the neck seemed stiff and painful when palpated, especially on the right side. Left lateroflexion was limited and painful. Electrical detection highlighted three points, two on the right and one on the left (Figure A.4). For the French, point 1 on the right in the cavum conchae corresponds to the cardio-pneumonic-enteric nucleus of the vagus nerve and in my opinion is frequently relevant in cases of allergy and defective metabolisms (the young woman's two grandmothers were both glucose intolerant and took oral antidiabetics). I often find that points 2 and 3, symmetrical and situated in the proximity of the posterior auricular groove (near the occipital point according to the Chinese) are relevant in cases of malocclusion and dysfunction of the temporomandibular joint. I used the extension and left lateroflexion movements of the lumbar spine as a reference for the Test. Point 1 was indifferent, point 2 was +, while point 3 gave a clear ++ response. I limited myself to puncturing point 3 and the patient was able to move freely and reported that the pain was reduced by 95%. Extraction of the needle caused moderate bleeding. At the next session the patient reported that she had been well all week and that she had continued to sleep with a high pillow without suffering from lower back pain in the early morning. Contracture of the neck muscles persisted and there was no change even during the third session. I suggested to the young woman that she consult a specialist and I saw her again together with Dr Renzo Ridi, an odontologist and expert in the correlation between dental occlusion and posture [12, 13, 14, 15].

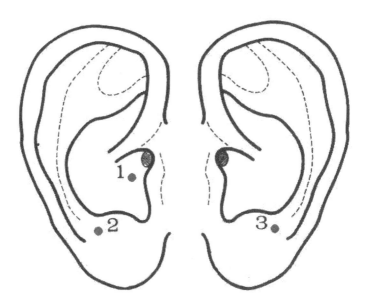

Figure A.4 Active Points Test on the ear in a case of cervicalgia with tension-headache in masseteric temporal regions

The stomatognathic examination showed a complete set of teeth and ample reconstructions of the occlusal surfaces of many posterolateral teeth with composite materials. Tendency to Class II, division 2 malocclusion (retroinclined upper central incisors). An orthopanoramic X-ray showed an impacted lower left wisdom tooth which was not painful when palpated and a bilateral flattening of the superior anterior part of the condyle. The patient, who had never undergone orthodontic therapy, exhibited a lateral deviation of the mandible to the left and a clicking in the left temporomandibular joint on opening the mouth. Palpation caused aching in the left temporomandibular joint, the medial temporalis muscles and the left lateral pterygoid muscle. A kinesiograph examination showed instability in the resting position of the mandible. The closing trajectory of the mandible showed posterior displacement; a steep anterior bite curve along the anterior wall. An electromyography using Myotronics' EM2 (Figure A.5) showed tension at rest in the submandibular muscles (DA), the left anterior temporalis muscle (TA), the right and left masseter muscles (Mm) and extreme tension in the sternocleidomastoid muscles (TP) bilaterally. Using the detector, I located point 3 which I had punctured during the previous sessions. I massaged this point with the tip of the palpeur, thus reducing tension in the SCM by 300% and in the submandibular and left anterior temporalis muscles by 50% (Figure A.6). These changes remained stable for the whole period of observation (30 minutes). It was suggested to the patient that she undergo Tens and acupuncture to normalise tension in the above-mentioned muscles. Once equilibrium in the muscles had been obtained with the mandible at rest, the patient would undergo bilateral isotonic stimulation of the elevator muscles of the mandible in order to record the muscle (not dental) closing point of the two arches of the jaw. Construction of the orthoptic device or neuromuscular bite would be based on this record (monitored by kinesiograph and EMG). The patient was also advised to improve the position of her head during sleep by using a pillow of the appropriate thickness. At the same time she was advised as to her overall posture in order to normalise myofascial contracture and to correct the misalignment of body segments.

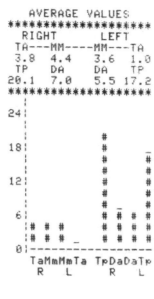

Figure A.5 Electromyography results before therapy

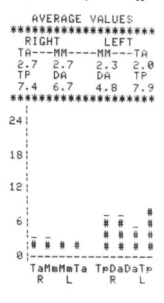

Figure A.6 Electromyography results after therapy

REFERENCES

[1]   Nogier, P.F.M. 'Traité d'Auriculothérapie'. Maisonneuve, Moulins-lès-Metz, 1969.

[2]   Roccia, L. 'Agopuntura auricolare cinese'. Edizioni Minerva Medica, Turin, 1978.

[3]   Li Su Huai 'Acupuncture Points: 2001'. China Acupuncture and Moxibustion Supplies, Taiwan, 1976.

[4]   Romoli, M. 'Alcune differenze dell'applicazione clinica tra auricoloterapia occidentale e orientale'. *Agop. e Tecniche di Terapia Antalgica*, 1, 19–39, 1986.

[5]   Jarricot, H. and Wong M. 'De l'Auriculothérapie'. *Meridiens*, 21, 85–137, 1973.

[6]   Jarricot, H. 'Projections viscérocutanées'. Atti delle Giornate Austro-FrancoItaliane, Turin, 31 May–2 June, 1974.

[7]   Romoli, M. 'Ear acupuncture and psychosomatic medicine: right–left asymmetry of acupoints and lateral preferences: Part II'. *Acupuncture & ElectroTherapeutics Research*, 1, 11–17, 1994.

[8]   Nogier, P.F.M. 'Complement des points réflexes auriculaires'. Maisonneuve, Moulins-lès-Metz, 1989.

[9]   Jarricot, H. 'Dermalgies réflexes viscérocutanées postérieures et organisation nouvelle du méridien principal de la Vessie'. *Meridiens*, 51, 97, 1980.

[10] Romoli, M., Poggiali, C., Candidi Tommasi, A., Lomi M., Soldi A. and Camurri F. 'Ispezione del padiglione auricolare e diagnosi di affezioni esofagogastroduodenali'. *Min. Riflessoter. e Laseter.*, 1, 7–14, 1987.

[11] Gianfranceschi, P., Gentile, A., Morales, R. and Giannotti C. 'Eliminazione delle intolleranze alimentari e miglioramento della performance muscolare'. Acts of the Medicina naturale a convegno. Milanofiori, 23–24 October, 1993.

[12] Ridi, R., Romoli, M. and Geri, L. 'Asimmetrie EMG e alterazioni dell'equilibrio occlusale in un caso di dismetria vera degli arti inferiori'. *Odontoiatria oggi*. Edizioni Piccin, 5 May, 1991.

[13] Ridi, R. 'Biomechanical and functional correlations between postural system and cranialmandibular region'. Records of the 8th Meeting of the European Society of Biomechanics, Rome, June 1992.

[14] Ridi, R. 'Relationship between occlusion and posture'. In 'Studies in health technology and informatics (vol. 5)', ed. A. Pedotti. IOS Press, Amsterdam, Oxford, Washington, Tokyo, 1993.

[15] Ridi, R. 'Nuovo approccio interdisciplinare allo studio delle correlazioni fisiopatologiche tra apparato craniomandibolare e sistema posturale con metodica di analisi strumentale integrata multifattoriale'. Acts of Congress 'Attività sportiva: analisi del movimento'. Association of Specialists in Sports Medicine at the University of Chieti, Arezzo, 1994.

ENDNOTES

1   Marcelli, S. 'Acupuncture Kinesiologic Test (AKT). Un test di chinesiologia per la scelta dei punti terapeutici nell'agopuntura, nell'auricolopuntura e nella mesoterapia'. Acts of the Medicina Naturale a Convegno – Assago – MI 23–24 October 1993. In the Abstracts of the 3° Congresso Nazionale Agopuntura E Tecniche Riflessoterapiche in Medicina Psicosomatica. *Giornale Italiano di Riflessoterapia ed Agopuntura* 5, 2. Edizioni Libreria Cortina, Turin, 1993.

2   Saudelli, G. 'La Touch Localization di Kinesiologia Applicata in Medicina Tradizionale Cinese: La medicina non convenzionale nella medicina non convenzionale'. Società Italiana di Agopuntura XIX Congresso Nazionale. Available at: www.meso.it/saudelli-akt.htm

3   Dujany, R. 'Kinesiologia Applicata'. Edizioni SCE, Milan, 1990.

4   Dujany, R. 'Teoria e impiego pratico della kinesiologia applicata'. Tecniche Nuove, Milan, 2000.

5   Barrett, S. www.quackwatch.com and Bolen, T. www.quackpotwatch.org/quackpots/quackpots/barrett.htm, accessed 11 April 2014

6   Kenyon, J. N. 'Tecniche moderne di Agopuntura'. Edizioni di red./studio redazionale, Como, 1985.

7   Voll R. 'La posizione topografica dei punti di misurazione dell'elettroagopuntura secondo Voll (EAV)', 3 vols. Guna, Milano, 1999.

8   Leonhardt, H. 'Fondamenti dell'elettroagopuntura secondo Voll'. Piccin Editore, Padua, 1982.

9   Newman Turner, R. 'Principi e pratica della Moxa. L'applicazione del calore ai punti di agopuntura. Guida alla terapia'. Edizioni di red./studio redazionale, Como, 1983.

10 Birch, S. and Ida, J. 'Japanese Acupuncture: A Clinical Guide'. Paradigm Publications, Taos, CA, 1998.

11 Cantoni, T. 'Anche i cinesi morivano, però... Introduzione alla teoria ed alla pratica dell'agopuntura tradizionale cinese'. Editoriale Jaka Book, Milan, 1982.

12 Faubert, A. 'Traité didactique d'Acupuncture Traditionelle'. Guy Trédaniel Éditeur, Paris, 1977.

13 Laurent, D., Léger, C., Timon, G. and Virol, M. 'Atlas didactique d'Acupuncture Traditionelle'. Guy Trédaniel Éditeur, Paris, 1978.

14 Low, R. 'The non meridial points of acupuncture. A guide to their location and therapeutic use'. Thorson Publishing Group, Wellingborough, 1988.

15 Maciocia, G. 'The Foundations of Chinese Medicine'. Churchill Livingstone, Edinburgh 1995.

16 Maciocia, G. 'La Clinica in Medicina Cinese'. Casa Editrice Ambrosiana, Milan, 1995.

17 Borsarello, J. 'Agopuntura'. Masson, Milan, 1990.

18 Marcelli, S. 'Agopuntura in tasca'. Nuova Ipsa Editore, Palermo, 1995.

19 Dumitrescu, I. F. 'Agopuntura scientifica moderna. Volume I. Progressi e prospettive'. Nuova Ipsa Editore, Palermo, 1992.

20 Marcelli, S. 'Omeopatia e terapie puntorie'. *Medicina Naturale*, March 1991. Tecniche Nuove, Milan.

21 Daniaud, J. 'I punti di Weihe'. Fratelli Palombi Editori, Rome 1988.

22 Pistor, M. 'Un défi thérapeutique: la mésothérapie'. Librairie Maloine S.A. Éditeur, Paris, 1974.

23 Multedo, J. P. 'Mésothérapie, la troisième circulation'. Les Hameau, Nouvelles Thérapies, Paris, 1985.

24 Multedo, J. P. and Marcelli, S. 'Manuale di Mesoterapia'. Edizioni Minerva Medica, Turin, 1990.

25 Ravily, J. 'Atlas Clinique de Mésothérapie'. PMI Publications Médicales Internationales, Boulogne, 1988.

26 Marcelli, S. '*Nappage* e Aspirazione. Una vecchia e nuova tecnica in agopuntura e mesoterapia'. Abstracts of the Terzo Congresso Nazionale Agopuntura E Tecniche Riflessoterapiche in Medicina Psicosomatica. *Giornale Italiano di Riflessoterapia e Agopuntura* 5, 2. Edizioni Libreria Cortina, Turin, 1993. Anche nella rivista Empedocle, 1. Nuova Ipsa Editore, Palermo, 1994.

27 Per approfondimenti sulla mesoterapia si veda anche: available at www. meso.it, accessed 11 April 2014.

28 Roccia, L. 'Insegnamenti di agopuntura', Edizioni Minerva Medica, Turin, 1978.

29 Cataldi, P. 'Neuralterapia'. Edizioni di red./studio redazionale, Como, 1981.

30 Marcelli, S. 'Medicine Parallele'. Edizioni Libreria Cortina, Turin, 1993.

31 Collegi di Medicina tradizionale di Pechino, Nanchino, Shanghai. 'Fondamenti di agopuntura e di Medicina Tradizionale Cinese'. Savelli Editori, Milan, 1982.

32 Melzack, R. and Wall P. D. 'Pain mechanisms: A new theory.' *Science*, 150, 171–9, 1965. Also see wikipedia 'Gate control theory of pain'. Redatto ad arte.

33 Wall, P. D. and Melzack R., 'On nature of cutaneous sensory mechanisms,' *Brain*, 85, 331, 1962.

34 Kandel, E. R., Schwartz, J. H. and Jessell, T. M. 'Principles of Neural Science', 4th ed., pp.482-486. McGraw-Hill, New York, 2000.

35 Ippocrate. 'Aforismi e Giuramento'. Tascabili Economici Newton, Rome, 1994.

36 Romoli, M. 'Agopuntura Auricolare'. UTET, Turin, 2003.

37 Bassani, L. 'Lombo-sacralgie. Approccio manuale e neuroriflesso alle affezioni lombo-sacrali e coccigee'. Edizioni Libreria Cortina, Turin, 1994.

38 Soulié De Morant, G. 'L'Acupuncture chinoise'. Maloine, Paris, 1972.

39 Sherrington, C. S. 'Experiments in examination of the peripheral distribution of the fibres of the posterior roots of some spinal nerves.' Communicated by Professor M. Foster, Sec. R. S. Received December 2, 1892.

40 Greenberg, S. 'The history of dermatome mapping'. *Arch. Neurol.*, 2003.

41 Balboni, G. C., Bastianini A. *et al.* 'Anatomia Umana'. Edi. Ermes, Milan, 1976, vol. III, p.278.

42 Gleditsch, J. M. 'Riflessoterapie. L'interpretazione unitaria di terapie orientali e occidentali.' Edizioni di red./studio redazionale, Como, 1991.

43 Geng Junying *et al.* 'Selecting the Right Acupoints. A Handbook on Acupuncture Therapy'. New World Press, Pechino, 1995.

44 Ross, J. 'Combinazione dei Punti di Agopuntura'. Casa Editrice Ambrosiana, Milan, 1999.

45 Gori, G. 'Il significato energetico dei punti di agopuntura'. San Marco Libri, Rimini-Venice, 1991.

46 Gori, G. and Bernabò, E. 'Agopunti' (CD Rom). myBox srl, Bologna, 2005.

47 Quaglia Senta, A. 'Il sistema simpatico in agopuntura cinese'. Edizioni Libreria Cortina, Turin, 1977.

48 Deadman, Al-Khafaji A. 'A brief discussion of the points of the Window of Heaven'. *Journal of Chinese Medicine*, 43, September 1993.

49 Académie de médecine traditionelle chinoise (Pékin) 'Précis d'acupuncture chinoise'. 5th ed. Édition Dangle, Saint-Jean-de-Bray,1977.

50 Nogier, P. 'Traité d'auriculothérapie'. Maisonneuve, Moulins-lés-Metz, 1969.

51 Bossy, J. 'Bases neurobiologiques des réflexothérapies'. Masson Éd., Paris, 1975.

52 Bourdiol, R. J. 'Réflexothérapie somatique'. Maisonneuve Éd., Metz, 1983.

53 Le Coz, J. 'Traité de Mésothérapie'. Masson, Paris, 2004.

54 Milani, L. 'Atti del X Congresso Nazionale della S.I.R.A.A'. L'Aquila, 8–9 September, 1994.

55 Streitberger, K. and Kleinhenz, J. 'Introducing a placebo needle into acupuncture research'. *The Lancet*, 352, Issue 9125, 364–365 K.

56 Nogier, P. 'Introduzione pratica all'auricoloterapia'. Edizioni Libreria Cortina, Turin, 1999, Édition SATAS sa. Bruxelles.

SUBJECT INDEX

AUTHOR INDEX

Made in the USA
Lexington, KY
23 January 2018